MAKE UP
YOUR LIFE

VICTORIA JACKSON

MAKE UP

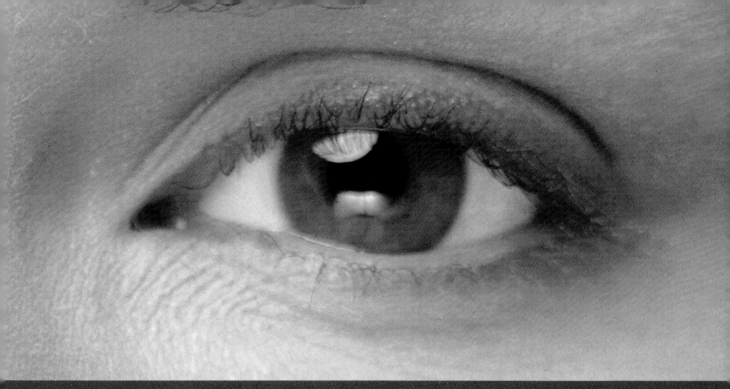

YOUR LIFE

Every Woman's Guide to the Power of Makeup

WITH ANDREA CAGAN

PHOTOGRAPHY BY DOUGLAS KIRKLAND

Cliff Street Books

An Imprint of HarperCollinsPublishers

DESIGNED BY JOEL AVIROM

DESIGN ASSISTANTS: MEGHAN DAY HEALEY AND JASON SNYDER

ILLUSTRATIONS BY JASON SNYDER

None of the celebrities pictured thoughout this book have endorsed Victoria Jackson or her products.

All photographs by Douglas Kirkland except: page 3 by Joan Lauren, page 148 by Just Us Photography, and pages 172–173 by Valerie Schaff

HarperCollins books may be purchased for educational, business, or sales promotional use. For information please write: Special Markets Department, HarperCollins Publishers Inc., 10 East 53rd Street, New York, NY 10022.

FIRST EDITION

Printed on acid-free paper

Library of Congress Cataloging-in-Publication Data has been applied for.

ISBN 0-06-019639-4

00 01 02 03 04 ❖/RRD 10 9 8 7 6 5 4 3 2 1

To my three Little Blessings,
Evan, Alexandra, and Jackson.
Your laughter, your spirit, and your innocence
continue to fill me with a peace and love
that I will cherish forever.

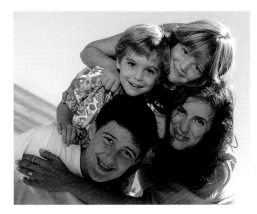

ACKNOWL

I AM ABSOLUTELY DELIGHTED to share my thoughts with you on the power of makeup. Without the wisdom and assistance of some very special people, this book would not exist.

I am especially grateful to my loving husband, Bill Guthy, who has continued to support me both personally and professionally. You're also a terrific dad. A special heartfelt hug to my son Evan, who underwent major surgery during the writing of this book. Thanks to my terrific daughter, Alexandra Rose, for managing to occupy yourself when your mother was busy. To my littlest one, Jackson William, you truly bring new meaning to the words, "a bundle of joy."

A very special thanks to my mother, Barbara, who always helps maintain order in my life. I'm so glad you told me to wash my face and put on some makeup during those formative years. I guess I listened, Mom. To my father, Mort, thanks for healing and staying healthy. I love you. And to my father, Sam, I'm so glad you're in my life. As for the rest of my family members, Mark, Dan, Andrea, Audrey, Nicole, I love you all dearly. Thanks for your constant encouragement.

A much needed thank you to Myrian and Raquel, who are so wonderful to my children. You give me the peace of mind to help me inspire others.

It has been a pleasure and a bonus to have made a friend and worked with such a terrific writer as Andrea Cagan. Your amazing capacity to translate my thoughts and words has truly made this a book I am very proud of. Through your reassuring smile and comforting words, I always knew I was in good hands.

It is an honor and a pleasure to work with Douglas and Françoise Kirkland once again. Douglas, your work always clearly and honestly portrays the natural beauty and captures the essence of each of the women you photograph. Your unbelievable body of work featured throughout this book is a testament to your generosity and abundance of talent. And to your beautiful wife, Françoise, you make every shoot enjoyable, adding so much style to each session.

EDGMENTS

Diane Reverand, my editor at HarperCollins Publishers, was so key to setting the tone and giving me the freedom to express my beliefs. Your positive attitude and belief in this book made the process a pleasure. To Jill Cohen at QVC Publishing, thank you for getting the ball rolling in the first place. Without your vision, this book would not have been the same. Many thanks to Joseph Montebello and Joel Avirom. Your inspired graphic designs and fabulous vision helped create a visual excitement on every page.

My gratitude to my agent, Jan Miller, for your persistence and your help in fulfilling my dream. Much appreciation goes to Guthy Renker Corporation for being terrific partners and advocates of this book. I will always be grateful for your support of my ideas and my products. Thank you to Gwinn Ioka for putting up with deadlines and just getting things done on time. And to Kareen Boursier, the book would not have been this beautiful without your touch.

A very special thank you to all the contributing voices: Vanna White, Judith Light, Marilu Henner, Rob Lowe, Garry Marshall, and Ali MacGraw, just to name a few. Your wisdom, grace, and generosity truly add to the spirit of this book.

Finally, to women the world over, whose positive spirits inspire me. Your faith in yourselves has encouraged and validated my belief that every woman is beautiful.

With love,

Victoria

CONT

ENTS

INTRODU

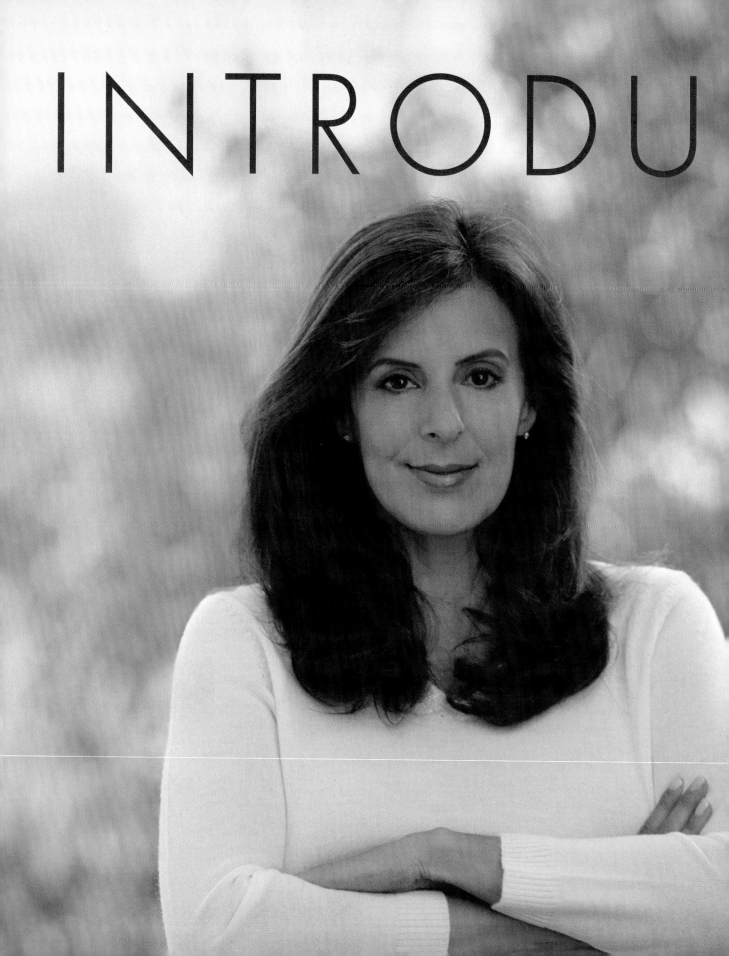

CTION

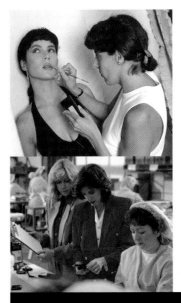

IT TOOK ME MORE THAN TWENTY YEARS to become an "overnight success" in the world of makeup—thirteen years as a makeup artist, ten years as Chairman of the Board of my own cosmetics company, and six successful infomercials. I've had the opportunity to watch makeup change women's lives and help them feel better about themselves from the big screen to the board room, from the dance floor to the bedroom. Among the various actors, models, news anchors, housewives, teachers, and corporate business executives who have been my clients, I've seen a common thread: makeup has the power to help instill confidence in people.

> *Women who live for the next miracle cream do not realize that beauty comes from a secret happiness and equilibrium within themselves.*
>
> *— Sophia Loren*

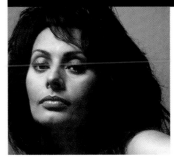

One of my earliest revelations as a makeup artist was how few beautiful women are able to accept their power and their own natural beauty. So many models and actresses have been programmed to hide behind heavy makeup. It used to be a big surprise when I chose not to change a woman's appearance dramatically. Rather, my goal was to make these beautiful women look like themselves, only better.

From this intention, my trademark, "No Makeup Makeup" was born. It's become a signature for my work. When you can accept that your natural features are already appealing (I know this isn't always easy), you can feel comfortable with or without makeup. Then you can learn to use makeup in the most natural way, making the most of your God-given beauty.

It could be that mascara makes you feel sexier. Maybe some lipstick and a little blush helps you feel more alive. You might be partial to using foundation, or maybe you love to bring out your eyes with eyeliner and some subtle shadow. Or maybe you like all of the above, and you're excited about a different method of application. The point is that makeup can empower you to feel more comfortable and confident about yourself. Then, you can put "how you look" behind you and participate in what matters most in life.

I believe there's a world of interesting and valuable experiences out there. Why waste time worrying about whether you look good enough? Isn't making something of yourself from the inside out a much worthier pastime than getting stuck on how somebody sees you? If you take a moment to broaden your knowledge about makeup, to learn to apply it in a simple, efficient, and effective way and feel good about how you look as a result, you can get on with the rest of your life. To me, feeling free is what power is all about, the gift I'd like to offer other women—the real reason I decided to write this book.

It's difficult to pinpoint the exact moment my interest in the power of makeup took hold. A deciding event did happen one afternoon, when I went wandering through the Max Factor museum near Hollywood Boulevard. I remember marveling at how ahead of his time he was. I fantasized about what this innovative man must have been thinking when he created new products that would change the face of makeup and of women forever. Inspired by what I saw, I went home and started mixing up my own concoctions in pots and pans in my garage.

My mom and me

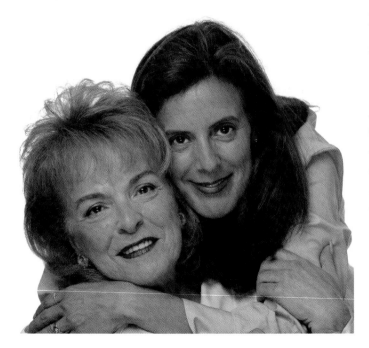

As far as hands-on training, my greatest teacher was my mother, although she had no idea. When I was facing any kind of challenge growing up, she used to say, "Victoria, wash your face, put on some makeup, get out there, and just do it." It was the old "fake it 'til you make it" concept. As simple as her advice was, I took it to heart. Today, as my company and my television career continue to expand, I still remember my mother's wise words. A little makeup combined with a positive attitude can go a long way.

For more than a decade, as makeup artist to some of the world's most gorgeous women, including Jackie Bisset, Brooke Shields, Rene Russo, Kate Capshaw, and Kathleen Turner to name a few, I've seen time and again, how makeup can build confidence in a woman. I recall a beautiful and prominent movie star arriving early at a shoot one

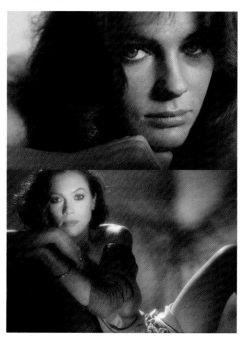

morning. Nervously sitting down in my makeup chair, she said she wasn't feeling all that well, and asked if I would make her up before her costar arrived. As I applied a light foundation and gave her some eyeliner, shadow, blush, and lipstick, she transformed into a different person. Finally, when the mascara went on, the outspoken sex symbol her public knew and loved was standing before me. As I watched her walk away with great confidence to greet the rest of the cast, I marveled at the extra bounce in her stride and how different she looked from when she'd sat down. Although she was a beautiful woman naturally, the truth was that she wasn't comfortable until she was wearing a little makeup. The outer change in her demeanor was dramatic, but the inner change was nothing short of a miracle.

As we women continue to gain more freedom and confidence in ourselves, I see attitudes toward makeup moving in a healthy direction. We're no longer following other people's ideas about what works for us and what doesn't. I'm relieved to see that we've stopped allowing the seasons to dictate our color palettes, that we've moved beyond that kind of rigid, boxlike thinking. These days, we're allowing our own creativity to dictate how we look in the moment. Most women instinctively know what looks best on them, anyway. We don't need anyone to tell us. Maybe we simply don't give ourselves enough credit. If we stop for a moment and take an honest look in the mirror, we can trust what our instincts tell us.

The future for women is promising. As we greet a brand-new millennium, we have brought with us a fusion of the fashion and makeup ideas of all the decades that came before. We are free to experiment, but there are certain basics that are timeless. For example, I doubt we'll ever go back to wearing clown cheeks or thick, pointy eyebrows. If, on a whim, we decide to wear dark eyes and light lips, or dark lips and light eyes, we can. It's okay to go to extremes or even to go without makeup altogether. With our hard-earned sense of freedom, we no longer need to paint masks on our faces. It's time to loosen up and have some fun, which is what we've been working

XIII

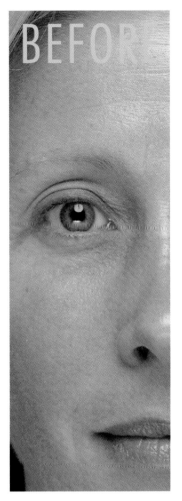

toward for a very long time. The more outspoken we become, the more we can appreciate what we have and who we are, as we allow more of ourselves to come through.

Fortunately, the desire to accentuate our natural beauty is being supported by new technologies in the manufacturing of cosmetics. In the ten years since I first created my Victoria Jackson cosmetic line, products have become much sheerer than they used to be. It's easy to create a more natural look. In 1989, looking natural was considered radical, and I was looked upon as a makeup rebel, breaking all the rules. The pendulum was swinging. We broke out of the fifties and into the sixties when makeup was about heavy lines. During the sixties and seventies, makeup was still pretty unnatural but the hippies went the other way—no makeup at all, take me or leave me, exactly as I am. As the pendulum swung back, we searched for a middle ground, which was all about discovering who we were, playing down what we liked the least, and enhancing what we liked the most.

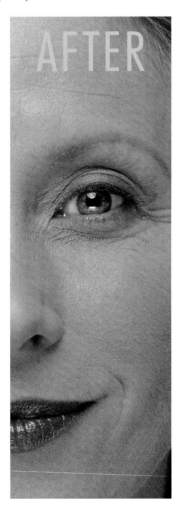

This is where we are today, and really, I'm not surprised. I've held a clear vision of a natural look in makeup from the day I took my little homemade concoctions to a chemist, who turned out to be one of the best in the business, and told him about the natural shades of foundation I envisioned. Having embraced the concept of "no makeup makeup" since I started my work as a makeup artist, my goals have remained the same. I want to help women not only to look natural, but also to feel better about themselves. From this concept, my cosmetic line was born.

In the pages to follow, my goal is much more than teaching you about makeup, although that is certainly a major focus. I'll be showing examples of "before and after," telling celebrity anecdotes, sharing portions of letters women have sent me throughout the years, and offering tips about how to use makeup to build on what you like about your face and play down what you don't. Along with dramatic photographs of makeovers, I'll also be explaining how to achieve the look you want in two, five, or ten minutes. It's my desire to offer simple techniques so that you can look good in a quick, clean, and efficient way. Who has two hours to get ready for a date or an event these days?

My greatest wish is to inspire you to be able to drop your insecurities and to allow your own power to shine through. *Make Up Your Life* is a "how-to" book, but I see it also as a why: why makeup makes a difference in your life, why you feel better when you wear it, and why being comfortable with the way you look ultimately will free you up.

Instead of using makeup as a way to hide, why not use it to celebrate who you're becoming? That's freedom—dropping the mask, taking a good look at what you have, and letting your beauty glow from the inside out. Don't you want to take pride in who you are? Instead of feeling self-conscious, wouldn't you rather be conscious of yourself?

It's my contention that when you look better, you feel better. When you feel better, you attract success. When you're successful, you have the self-esteem to take on more challenges and to dedicate your life to a higher purpose. That's the way you can make up the life you want, the real power of makeup.

Victoria Jackson
March 2000

MAKE UP
YOUR LIFE

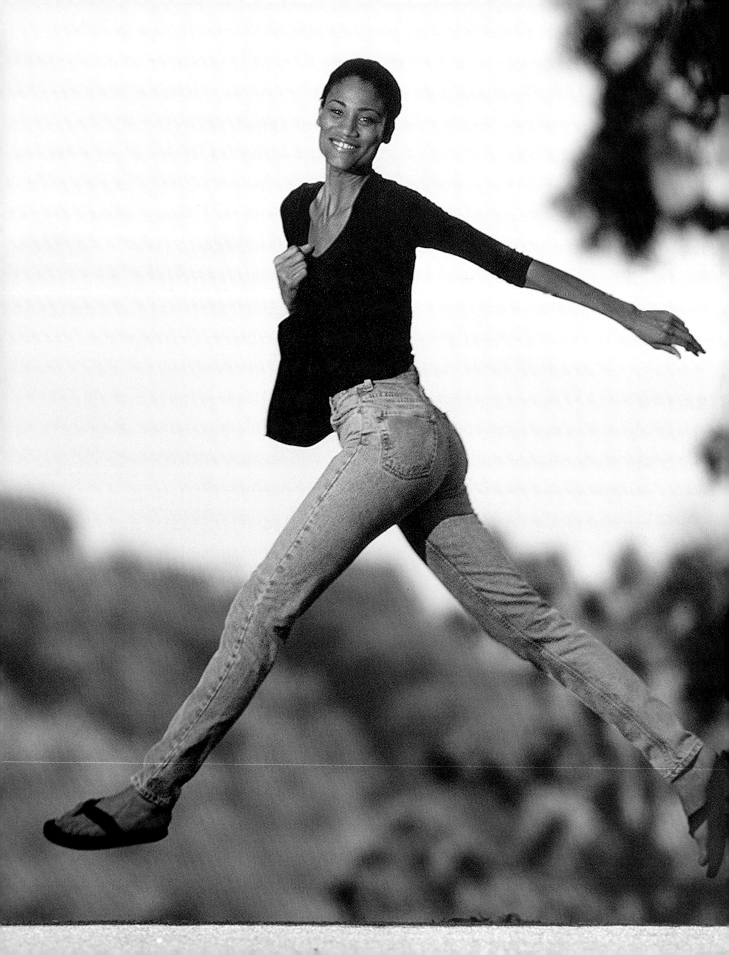

1: MAKE UP YOUR LIFE

FEELING BEAUTIFUL Have you ever passed a woman walking down the street and suddenly realized that everybody was looking at her, including you? At second glance, she may not be all that beautiful, at least not in classical terms. She may not have "perfect" features or be as thin or exotic-looking as the fashion model gracing the cover of the magazine you're holding. And yet, she exudes an enviable confidence, a certain indescribable something that turns heads.

I bet you think I'm going to suggest it's all in the makeup. After all, this is a book about makeup, I have my own cosmetic company, and it's the logical thing for me to say. Right? The truth is I don't believe that makeup has all that much to do with it, at least not directly. This woman draws attention, not because she has on a luscious shade of lipstick, magnificently long eyelashes, or the perfect blush to her cheeks. In fact, she may be not wearing makeup at all, her nose may be crooked, her lips uneven, and her complexion may not be perfect. And yet, she attracts your attention.

It's her self-assured step, the grace with which she moves her body, the way she holds her head as if she has a special secret that

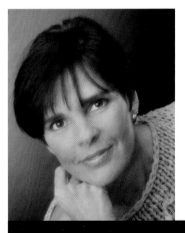

When I do the serious work of getting to know who I really am — and then live by my principles and not the opinion of others, I have self-confidence. Nothing external can really do that for me.

— Ali MacGraw

makes her feel great about being alive. She may or may not be as mysterious as she looks, but one thing is sure: The way she feels about herself from the inside affects the way she looks on the outside. This is the origin of real beauty, and whether makeup detracts from it or enhances its essence, is all in the way you use it.

The mystery that a beautiful woman exudes is not a black magic spell, but it's magic, nonetheless, the same kind that happens when you recognize your own natural beauty, revel in it, and allow it to shine wherever you go. When the USA women's soccer team won the World Cup last year, the team members did most of their victory publicity, including TV and magazine spreads, without a drop of makeup on their faces. And yet, everyone, men and women alike, commented on how beautiful they all looked. They became instant role models for young girls and women everywhere, just because they exuded the kind of self-assurance that made them appear beautiful.

The lesson here is that you don't have to be a classic beauty to look or feel fresh and pretty, to have a wonderful and satisfying life, or even to be considered beautiful. You don't have to go to the gym every day, wear expensive clothes, or be made-up perfectly every time you leave the house. Beauty begins much deeper than at the end of a magic wand of mascara or a compact of luscious red lip color. These items can all contribute to a great look and to an overall sense that a woman is pulled together, but beauty is something else altogether.

Beauty has eluded description since Venus de Milo was sculpted. If you examine photographs of models or celebrities and remove the hair and clothes, you'll discover that their attractiveness is not dependent upon a sexy dress, an oval-shaped face, or a

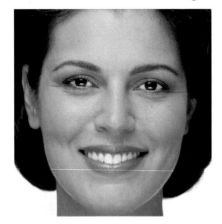

pot of eye shadow. It comes from an attitude that exudes self-acceptance and the celebration of being alive.

When you approach your life with enthusiasm, focusing on the wonder and the fun, you become more conscious of your vibrancy which allows your natural beauty to shine through. Remember that old cliché, "Beauty is in the eyes of the beholder?" I'd like to change it to, "Beauty is in the way we hold ourselves."

THE REAL YOU Living by misconceptions about beauty, makeup, and being a woman in general, can be hazardous to your health. Anytime you get locked into believing in an outdated philosophy, you run the risk of stagnation. We all see ourselves differently from the way others do, so stop comparing yourself to supermodels. Rather, appreciate them as beautiful women, and use them as templates to create the look that best suits your own individuality.

When you start believing that you can be or do anything, the possibilities are staggering. Today, the world of beauty is an empty page waiting to be filled with new ideas and philosophies. Why get stuck in the past? Instead of trying to conform to unrealistic guidelines about beauty, how about changing them to create a new beauty reality?

It's a good sign for women that there are other product lines besides mine that have adopted the natural look. This is happening because we women are demanding it. We're healthier than we used to be, we eat better, we work out, our skin looks better, and we have very little time to prepare for the day. We're not interested in looking overly done, and even if we were, who has the time? Thank heavens we don't draw fake beauty marks on our faces, manicure our eyebrows down to thin little lines, or paint our cheeks to look as if we're permanently blushing. We're starting to accept the way we look and to put our best selves forward, not an image of somebody else. There's an Australian aboriginal saying, "The more you know, the less you need." It's time to look in the mirror, know who you are, and understand how you can realize your greatest beauty potential with the least effort.

Remember that you are free to wear your makeup anyway you like. I'm not suggesting that it's not okay to play. Feel free to have fun and enjoy yourself, that's all part of the joy of being a woman. At the same time, keep in mind that rainbow eyes and the kind of bizarre costumes that models wear in magazine layouts or on the runways are not for the real world. These looks are like art statements, and they should be viewed and enjoyed with that in mind. Never forget that the "real you" is the best look you have. Learn to know it, love it, enhance it, and flaunt it. You are your greatest asset.

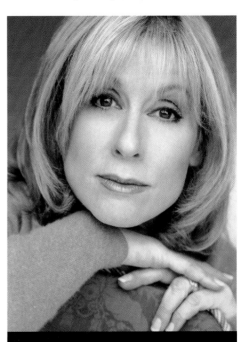

Victoria understands that it isn't makeup that is important, but that makeup really supports what is important, and that is the way we feel about ourselves and the implications of the ways we present ourselves to the world.

—Judith Light

AGELESS BEAUTY Nowhere did I see the "eye of the beholder" more elegantly illustrated than when I had the good fortune to work with movie-star legend, Bette Davis, more than a decade ago. Shortly before she died, I was hired to make her up for a print campaign for a TV movie. I felt privileged to have the opportunity to meet such an extraordinary and talented woman. When I began applying foundation to her deeply wrinkled skin, she stopped me, gently took my hand, and said, "Honey, don't bother trying to cover those wrinkles. I've earned every one of 'em."

When I stepped back, I saw her ageless beauty shining through, the magnificence she had embraced in herself. What a revelation! This woman, in her eighties, was comfortable with who she was, as well as proud of her experience and her age. In fact, she had so completely accepted her lines and wrinkles as a symbol of a life well-lived, she wanted to flaunt them!

I was inspired. I'll always remember her apart from others who were more concerned with concealing their flaws than revealing their strengths. They may have been more perfect-looking than Ms. Davis, but when it came to dazzle, this octogenarian outshone every one of them. All because of the way she felt about herself.

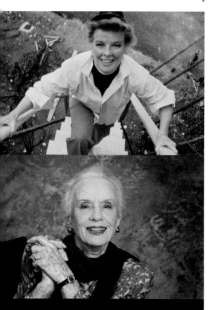

We are born with one face, but, laughing or crying, wisely or unwisely, eventually we form our own.

— Coco Chanel

I took the lesson I learned from Bette Davis to heart when I was on my way to shoot my first infomercial, more than ten years ago. I felt extremely insecure, because I'd spent years making other people beautiful for the camera, and now it was my turn. I just didn't know if I measured up. I wondered, What is a Chairman of the Board of a cosmetics company supposed to look like? Or sound like? Beverly Sassoon, a very glamorous friend of mine, who also had her own cosmetics company, had the right look. I felt far from it.

When we pulled up to the shoot in a limo (to which I was not accustomed), I noticed that the streets were blocked off. "Oh, there's a shoot going on," I thought to myself. "I wonder who it is." I realized it was for me, that they'd blocked off the streets for my infomercial. Then I was really scared. This was a huge deal, and the pressure was building. When I walked onto the set, the walls had been decorated with my logo, VJ, framing a variety of blown-up covers and photographs I'd worked on. If someone had run out and said, "Victoria Jackson, this is your life!" I wouldn't have been the slightest bit surprised.

As I tried to swallow the lump in my throat, the producer brought me over to the French cinematographer, a rather stern and imposing man. He stared at me for a moment and said in a thick

Grandma Bertha Carson

accent, "There are two kinds of women, those with great beauty and those with great brains. You," he said, "are a woman with great brains."

Had he just called me a dog? We were standing in a group of people who were watching me carefully to see how I'd react. I was devastated, but I summoned the part of me that rises to adversity. I looked him right in the eye and said rather proudly, "So, it's lucky for me I'm in the best hands, because I know you're going to make me look absolutely beautiful."

As much as it had hurt at the time, his sharp comment was a gift. It made me recognize that this was my life, this was my moment, and nobody could take it away. All I needed was to accept my own beauty, believe in my personal power, and the rest would follow. I went out there and did the best job I'd ever done, just to show them all, and more importantly to show myself, who I really was. I know Bette Davis would have approved!

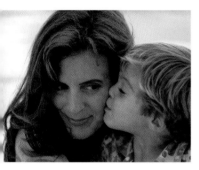

Jackson and me

BRIGHTENING YOUR OUTLOOK Makeup won't make love happen or guarantee that you'll get the job, but it can be great fun, a small indulgence that can boost your spirits. Although wearing makeup won't make you rich and famous or guarantee that promotion, using it to enhance your natural beauty is one of the positive aspects of being a woman. Of course, we need to be realistic about the gifts that makeup can bring us. It won't make you love yourself or de-age you or miraculously remove wrinkles from your skin. Wrinkles don't just fade away. Self-love is a hard-earned reward we give to ourselves with work and patience.

Although makeup won't change the circumstances of your life, it will change the way you view yourself. Seeing a bright face looking back at you from the mirror is uplifting and an enjoyable experience. We sometimes forget that we're always capable of raising our own self-esteem, no matter how we happen to feel on any given day. I've had times in my life when I felt down for one reason or another. Adding a little color to my face and some mascara to my eyelashes brightened my outlook. The makeup didn't change the external situation. It just gave me an added edge so I could face my life in a more positive way. Ultimately, putting on some makeup allowed me to put my appearance behind me, as I went on to face the challenges of the day with a little more self-confidence.

A well-respected doctor told me there is actually a medical diagnosis called "the positive makeup sign." When a woman is recovering from a serious illness, the day she puts on her makeup and brushes her hair indicates the fact that she's starting to heal. This signal demonstrates the connection between how a woman looks and her health.

Several years ago, I sponsored what I called "A Day of Beauty" at the Cedars-Sinai Comprehensive Cancer Clinic for a group of women who'd been physically ravaged by chemotherapy. For these women, literally everything was out of control. Some of them had lost their eyebrows, their skin was reddened, their faces were bloated, and they could hardly recognize themselves. As I showed them how to brighten up their faces and to hide some of the redness and other side effects, they became uplifted. By gaining a small degree of control over how they looked, they experienced a discernible difference in their spirits. For a short while, their difficult lives had become slightly more bearable.

Always remember — the best use of makeup is not to change the way you look. Rather, highlighting your natural features will confirm how nice they are to begin with. Projecting your natural beauty can be empowering, and makeup can provide an affordable and effective tool to do just that. People who feel positive about who they see in the mirror have more success in life than those who don't. And they also have a lot more fun!

MYTH:

SOME WOMEN CAN WEAR THE "NATURAL LOOK"
AND OTHERS CAN'T.

REALITY:

EVERY WOMAN HAS HER OWN NATURAL BEAUTY.

I've never met a woman who wasn't beautiful in her own special way with her own individual style. Once you know yours, you can enhance it with a minimum of makeup and end up looking terrific. It just takes some self-esteem, a desire to move beyond misconceptions, and a little makeup knowledge.

Instead of trying to live up to images set by other people, it's time to look in the mirror and see the truth about yourself. This is where good friends come in. If you have trouble seeing beyond your own preconceptions, perhaps a friend can help you be objective. When you really believe that less is more, and you trust yourself enough to live it, you'll discover beauty you never knew you had!

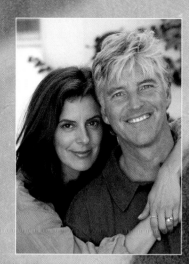

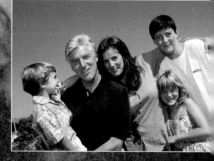

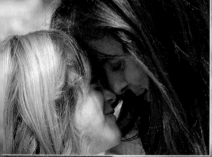

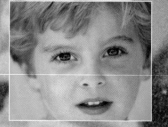

The family album

2: READING YOUR OWN SUCCESS STORY

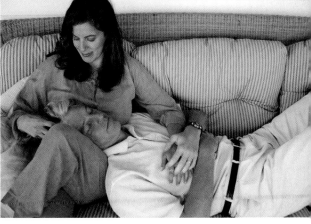

DREAMS AND GOALS I've always been a dreamer. Even at three years old, I had a sense of wonder and I questioned everything. I thought I wanted to be a teacher, so I could get up in front of people and talk—about what, I have no idea. It just appealed to me to be center stage and to have people paying attention to me. I also wanted a husband, babies, and plenty of chocolate ice cream—all age appropriate dreams.

Years later, when I was a teenager helping my friends put on their makeup, I had already decided that I wanted to be involved in the beauty business, one way or the other. It wasn't until the early eighties, though, while teaching at UCLA, that I really began to manifest my dream by creating my first product.

Do you remember your dreams and take them with you throughout the day? I'm talking about your daydreams, those elusive ideas that come to you in the shower or on the freeway that you hardly dare to talk about. C'mon, we all have them. What about those secret goals and desires that seem so unreachable, you either ignore them or pass them off as nothing more than fantasy? Or can you see yourself in extremely rewarding, real-life situations that bring you satisfaction and abundance? The answers to these questions are important, because your dreams and goals will determine the quality of your future. I always say that if you don't have dreams, you'll have nightmares. When women ask me how I parlayed an idea about foundation into a multi million dollar cosmetics company, the answer is straightforward: I held on to my dream.

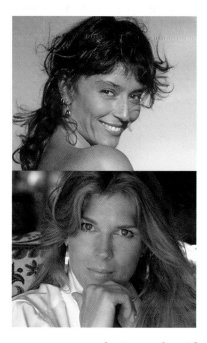

BREAKING NEW GROUND
For my first cosmetics job, behind the counter at Bullock's department store in Westwood many years back, I remember spending a good half hour every morning applying "the look" they wanted me to have. My days behind the counter were numbered because being "all dolled up" didn't feel good to me, so how could I sell that concept to other women? I learned quickly that women didn't want someone to sell them a ton of makeup or a bill of goods, anyway. What they really wanted was honesty, someone they could trust to give them real guidance as to what would make them look and feel better.

When I couldn't find a foundation that would capture the beauty of a woman without her looking heavily made-up, I realized it was time to go into business for myself. In fact, I was still a novice in the

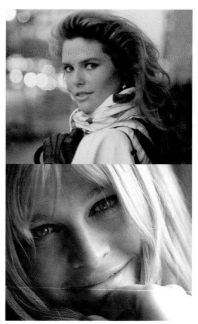

business when I first decided to have my own foundation manufactured. My goal was to create a product that would even out skin tones and conceal flaws while allowing a woman to look and feel as if she was not wearing makeup at all. At the time, I remember creating neutral-based shades of foundation, as in more natural to a real skin tone. People used to call me a pioneer in the cosmetic industry, which made me laugh as I imagined myself in my little covered wagon, touting the "no makeup makeup" concept to disbelieving customers. And yet, I suppose I was ahead of my time, since I was the first person ever to sell makeup successfully on television.

The idea behind my products and their application has remained the same over the years: spending the least amount of time to create a great look and appear as if you're not wearing makeup. I've always been less concerned about covering and concealing, and more focused on allowing the natural tone of the skin to shine through.

By the way, the shift hasn't been automatic for everyone. Using lighter makeup is something we all have had to get used to. It was easier to wear minimal makeup when I was in my twenties, than today, when I'm in my forties. I obviously wear more makeup now than I used to, but I still keep the "natural" concept close to my heart, using it to guide me in my personal daily makeup application. I want to be able to create a wonderful face for myself, look like me, and have it feel good, all at the same time. If it feels odd and different for you, give yourself time to reframe your attitude and your vision of yourself. You'll be glad you did.

> *As an ex-makeup artist, I have experienced the extraordinary power of just a little makeup, applied correctly. Well-applied makeup highlights a woman's face, charging every facial feature with a vibrant energy.*
>
> *— Ole Henriksen,*
> *skin care expert*

VISUALIZING SUCCESS

Before I ever knew I'd have my beautiful family, I was busy working on little old ladies with blue hair in beauty college. That was when I discovered my love for makeup. One thing flowed into the next, as I went from school to working in a department store cosmetic counter and offering free makeup services to photographers so I could build my portfolio. My big break finally happened when I got hired (yes, it was actually a paying job) as a makeup artist for a *People* magazine cover with Larry Hagman, the star of *Dallas*, the top-rated TV show at the time. One cover led to another, until I became a top makeup artist for magazines, TV, and film.

The point is that I had become a successful multi-media makeup artist, and yet, I couldn't shake a more compelling passion—to own a cosmetics company. I yearned to create products that would perform better than what was available, but getting there was not a smooth ride. There were the well-meaning "friends" who adamantly pointed out why it wouldn't work. "People aren't going to buy cosmetics from an infomercial," they droned. "It's never been done before because women have to see the colors with their own eyes and feel the textures. It simply won't fly. You're wasting time and money."

Granted, it took a great deal of time, but I didn't have to worry about wasting money, because I didn't have any. Against this backdrop of discouraging voices, I put

11

together my own limited partnership. My task was to raise fifty-thousand dollars by selling twenty-five shares of stock in a very short period of time. I sold eighteen shares before I reached an impasse—so close and yet so far. The deadline came and went and I didn't make it. With my tail between my legs, I returned my backers' investments, thanking them for their belief in me, but I felt embarrassed and defeated. I had reached the first major fork in the road to success.

I faced two choices—give up or keep going. I kept going, placing my larger dream on the back burner and continuing to develop my product line. I was my entire company and my one and only employee. Using my garage for an office, I sectioned it off into an art department, a marketing department, a portion dedicated to product development, and another to correspondence, if I could only get some. (I try to remember this when the stacks of mail in front of me are so overwhelming, that I don't know how I can possibly answer them all.)

After I took an order on the phone, I'd put on my delivery girl hat, flip up the huge garage door, and slide it back to get outside, which worked wonders on my biceps! Then I'd return from a delivery and get right back on the phone to generate more sales. At the time, I had my foundation in only three beauty supply stores, but I maintained a white-knuckled grip on my vision of success.

When I first came out with my new foundation shades, I had no extra money for fancy packaging. I remember taping my name around the "no frills" little round jars, and putting them on my nightstand. I'd drop off to sleep each night visualizing massive amounts of product pouring off of conveyor belts. In fact, I'd pretend to be on *The Oprah Winfrey Show*, reading my own success story, telling the world all about my journey and what I had accomplished.

"Victoria," Oprah would say in my mind, "tell us how you created such a successful business."

Smiling in the dark in my bed, I would recount to an invisible television audience some of the trials and tribulations that I'd overcome. I'd imagine I was reading a news article that described me as married with a few wonderful children, a multimillion dollar cosmetic company, and of all things—a book of my own. Then I'd take the feeling of success into my dreams. The next morning, I'd wake up renewed, and head back into my garage/office to start all over again.

As it turned out, returning the money to my investors was the best thing that ever could have happened. If I'd created the limited partnership and sold all the stock, I would not have been able to sign the contracts for my infomercial since I would have been otherwise obligated. What appeared to be my greatest obstacle and failure, was in truth, a total blessing.

The important thing to remember is that success takes time and an iron will. There are going to be obstacles and small failures along the way. It's all part of playing the game. Every mother knows the challenges of balancing a career, motherhood, and a relationship. I certainly stopped believing in the myth of being "Supermom" and "Superwoman" a long time ago. I don't do everything right, and my kids never miss an opportunity to point that out. My advice is to just do the best you can as you go along, and remember that dwelling on your disappointments will get you nowhere fast. Pain and sacrifice are true tests of character, and they always pop up along the path to success. Learn to zig and zag at the appropriate times, hold on to your passion, and you're certain to find what you're looking for.

WORKING WITH YOUR LIMITATIONS
Several years after I'd become Chairman of the Board of Victoria Jackson Cosmetics, I got that call from Oprah Winfrey's producers to be on her show. She was doing a segment on women who had made it against the odds, and they wanted me for the leading story. I thought I'd finally made it—until I had to confront a big problem—I don't fly.

You see, when I was a teenager, I was the victim of a violent crime, which left me with traumatic claustrophobia. I could have driven or taken a train to Chicago for the taping, but I kept fooling myself into believing that I could make the flight. The day before the flight was scheduled, I really had to face myself. Should I attempt to get on the plane and run the risk of laying more trauma over what I already had, or should I do the kind thing for myself and pass? I decided to accept my limitations rather than risk damaging myself further, but I was too embarrassed to tell the truth. I came up with an excuse, I can't even recall what I told the producers, but the upshot was that they did the show without me.

The day it aired, I cried while I watched somebody else sit in "my" seat and tell her story instead of mine. I learned that day, that no matter how successful you become or how good you are at visualizing and manifesting your dreams, there will always be challenges you can't foresee. It's back to the immortal words of my mother—pick yourself up, wash your face, put on some makeup, and turn your failures into a small chapter of your large success story.

To this day, I still dream about the Oprah show, and I believe in my heart that you'll be seeing me on the air one of these days—maybe even to promote this book. In the meantime, I continue working on myself and my company, learning to accept my limitations, and visualizing the day I'll be free of this fear.

MAKING IT WORK
Before I created my company, I was accustomed to being in the background and making someone else look fabulous. Center stage was for other people, not me, and I often arrived at a film or TV shoot, deliberately wearing no makeup at all, just to make the star feel more secure.

Most people don't know that I'm in business with my husband, which carries with it a unique set of difficulties. Try sitting across the dinner table from the very person with whom you were butting heads just hours earlier. In my case, it's important that we both leave our business at the door, and show up as parents to our children and partners to each other. This has helped me be a better businesswoman, as I've had to excel in managing my time and my emotions. The boardroom has been a great teacher for me.

Since negotiations are about integrating the needs and opinions of more than one person, when I'm in a business meeting, I put myself in the shoes of the other people around the table. If someone is lobbying for a particular point, I try to see it from his or her point of view, as well as from my own. When you're self-made and have worn every possible business hat along the way, you have a pretty broad perspective. It's something I haven't lost, and I make it a point never to talk down to anyone.

Nowadays, I'm not nervous in the boardroom the way I used to be. There's always some stage fright, but I've learned to label it "excitement" instead of fear or nervousness, and use it to my advantage. As long as I know what my goals are, I can enjoy being center stage and taking control of the room. By the way, these days, if I get an idea and a line forms at my door to tell me why it won't work, I figure I'm on the right track.

THE ENTREPRENEURIAL SPIRIT
Women everywhere want to know how they can do what I do. All I can say is that in order to be an entrepreneur, you have to reach really deep down and see what you're made of. You need to get clear about your message, feel connected to it, and then put it out there for all the world to see. Nothing supports this more than taking the focus off of yourself and giving something back.

Some of the most rewarding moments in my career have been while I was helping women with cancer. Whenever I spent time with them and showed them how to smile again and feel beautiful for the first time in months or years, I walked away both humbled and inspired. Helping others has been vital to my character development. Many of us need to discover, as I did, that success is ultimately based upon more than just making money and having a great wardrobe. Those things are wonderful and you should certainly enjoy them, but true success is measured in spirit. In 1997, when I was named Woman of the Year by the Los Angeles County Commission of Women for my self-esteem work in LA County prisons, it only helped to grow my business and make me feel better about myself. Helping less fortunate people and reaching out to those who helped you along the way completes the circle of success.

As I look at photos of my family and remember the struggles of trying to work it out, in retrospect, it was all worth it. The problems dissolve into the background and the joys outweigh the lean years. I wouldn't trade it for anything, even the times when I felt like nobody understood or appreciated me.

Keep in mind that when you're starting out, the very notion of being underpaid and underappreciated means you're paying your dues. Complaining will only move your success further out of reach. Instead, if you reach out and give of your time and energy to others while you hold on to your dream, you just may find yourself in the right place at the right time. Believe me, if it happened to me, it can happen to you.

MYTH:
BEAUTY EQUALS SUCCESS.

REALITY:
BEAUTY DOES NOT GUARANTEE SUCCESS.

People think that extraordinarily beautiful women have everything. It isn't true. Marilyn Monroe was one of the most beautiful women in the world, and she took her own life. Beauty does not guarantee success—or anything else for that matter. Beauty is just beauty. Success is something else altogether. The two can be completely separate or they can show up in one package, but one does not automatically ensure the other.

Successful women, beautiful or not, do seem to radiate a certain glow from within. That's because they *feel* successful and it reflects on the outside. Consider First Lady Hillary Rodham Clinton. She is by no means a classic beauty, but her sense of inner strength and her personal convictions add to her attractiveness.

3: MIRROR, MIRROR

ACCEPT YOURSELF Accepting yourself is the most important step along the path to feeling beautiful. This sounds easy enough, but with the media on a mission, it seems, to convince us that we need to be different from the way we are, it's a daunting task to feel good about ourselves these days, just as we are. With so much programming coming at you from all sides, both subliminal and in your face, it's hard to look at yourself honestly and appreciate your most wonderful assets. Instead, women have become accustomed to picking themselves apart, focusing incessantly on what's wrong. I sometimes fall prey to this negative thinking. It's sad to waste time obsessing about how you look, instead of learning to evaluate yourself with an honest and loving eye, and then to cash in on what's right. In fact, this very point has been one of my major motivations in writing about beauty.

AU NATUREL Vanna White is a gorgeous woman and a famous TV personality who feels so good about herself, she's comfortable allowing millions of home viewers to see her *au naturel*, with no makeup on her face. We're friends, and I wanted her to be in my latest infomercial, but I was apprehensive to ask. I knew she liked my products because she'd been using them for quite a while, but I wanted to show her in a "before

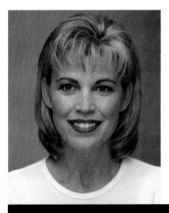

You don't have to put on a full face of makeup. It depends on the time of day and where you're going. I prefer a light touch of makeup for daytime use and I add a little more for the evenings.

— Vanna White

and after" makeup application. That meant she'd have to appear on TV with no makeup at all. I didn't know how she'd feel about that. To my delight, she agreed without hesitation. Vanna was so at ease during the shooting, it inspired me to be just as relaxed. The upshot is that we both appeared without makeup in "before and after" demonstrations, and we both felt great about it.

Ali MacGraw is another radiantly beautiful woman who's as comfortable in her natural state as she is when she's made-up. These are the women we can fashion ourselves after, women who make up their own lives and understand the power of makeup.

RESPECT YOURSELF Beauty for the new millennium is a great deal more than good looks and physical attributes. Beauty involves honesty and self-respect, the natural qualities you were born with. Who you are on the inside shows on your face, and so does your self-confidence, your accomplishments, and your kindness. However you see yourself right now, you have unlimited potential to feel good about yourself and your looks, and to appreciate your God-given gifts. If you retrain yourself to respect who you are and act accordingly, you can concentrate on what's important in life, instead of what you see in the mirror.

Try an experiment with me. Wash off all your makeup, (yes, every bit, mascara and all), and look in the mirror. Let the real "you" show. If you see this as a scary proposition, you're probably in the habit of looking at yourself negatively. So many women are accustomed to giving themselves negative messages, which creates a distorted picture of who they are. The truth is that all women are beautiful, God made you that way, and your task is to see your best qualities first.

All women are beautiful. Makeup helps them believe they are.
— *Garry Marshall, director*

Do you need some help? If it's too hard to see yourself in a respectful and beautiful light, it may be time to call in a trusted friend. Ask her about your best features. A good friend's opinion, which is apt to be kinder than your own, might get you on the right track. Then you can take it from there. The idea is to be realistic, to find out who you are, and then to accept yourself.

You may be thinking, "I look at myself every day. What's the big deal?" True, you may be used to looking at yourself in the mirror, but up until now, you may not really have seen yourself. When you stop long enough to really look, you may be amazed at what you find. As women in a fast-moving and, at times, unforgiving world that shuns aging and idolizes youth, we all share the same insecurities. It's shocking to discover that even the most stunning women in the world rarely consider themselves beautiful. I remember a girlfriend reading me an interview with Michele Pfeiffer, who said she thought she looked like a duck. Distraught, my

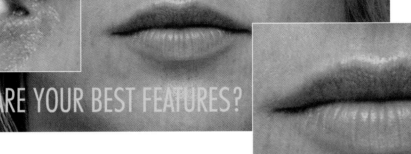

WHAT ARE YOUR BEST FEATURES?

friend turned to me and said, "If she looks like a duck, I wonder what we look like?"

Assuming you're willing to discover your own beauty, when you look in the mirror what do you see? Remember, be kind. Don't list all the things that are wrong first. Women are always pointing out to me what they consider their problem areas—dark circles under the eyes, a thin bottom lip, undefined cheekbones. The list goes on and on. It almost never happens that a woman tells me, "Victoria, you know I really like the way my eyes look," or, "I love my mouth, I have a great full top lip."

What if you saw what you liked first? Wouldn't life feel kinder? Of course, you need to see all of it, the negatives and the positives, but you can retrain yourself to see the positive aspects first. These are the features that you like and want to enhance. If you start with what's right, you can look at makeup the way I do. Rather than using it solely to correct what's wrong, I appreciate makeup as a miraculous tool to enhance what's right.

> *Comparing myself to other women can create a negative, competitive feeling. When I take the time to eat well, exercise, spend real time with my children and my husband . . . when I meditate and remember to breathe, I end up being happier with who I am and can really enjoy the company of other women. In my field, there are too many extraordinary looking women. I'd never be able to leave the house if I compared myself to them.*
>
> — *Julie Carmen, actress*

Very few women appreciate their own loveliness. I'm too pale, you might say, or I'm too dark, too crooked, too pointy, too fat, too thin (well, hardly ever), too tall, too short, or just too much *you*. Instead of celebrating individuality, women have been taught to strive for what I call "cosmetic ad perfection," heading for the cookie cutter image instead of accentuating their own particular allure. All too often, I see women hiding their special features because they're different. If they don't have oval faces, almond eyes, and thin, straight noses, they think they aren't pretty.

Comparing yourself to some unattainable image of beauty is a surefire way to miss the special qualities of your own face. Consider Cindy Crawford's mole over her lip and Barbra Streisand's nose. These women have learned to accept what they have so completely, these "flaws" are their most outstanding features. Why not celebrate your individuality instead of wasting time and money attempting to achieve "cosmetic perfection?" You won't get there anyway, and in the meantime, you'll be busy hiding your magnificence beneath a ton of unnecessary makeup.

There is no makeup that will transform your face into someone else's. What gave you the idea that another person's cheekbones would look better on you than your own? A highly respected fashion photographer told me that a very successful modeling agency recently opened for beautiful women with features that don't fall into the classic interpretation of perfection. We've come a long way in expressing our individuality and having it appreciated. It's a good time for women, there's room for so much more than there used to be. Let's take advantage of it.

The best plan is to get rid of whatever is camouflaging your individual beauty. I'm not suggesting you get rid of your makeup altogether. If I thought makeup was of no use, I wouldn't be writing this book. What I am doing is urging you to take a good look at yourself, accept what you see, and then play with what you've got.

When you ask the legendary question, "Mirror, mirror, on the wall, who's the fairest of them all," let the answer be, "All women are fair, including me." It's time to drop the judgments and find out how special and beautiful you really are.

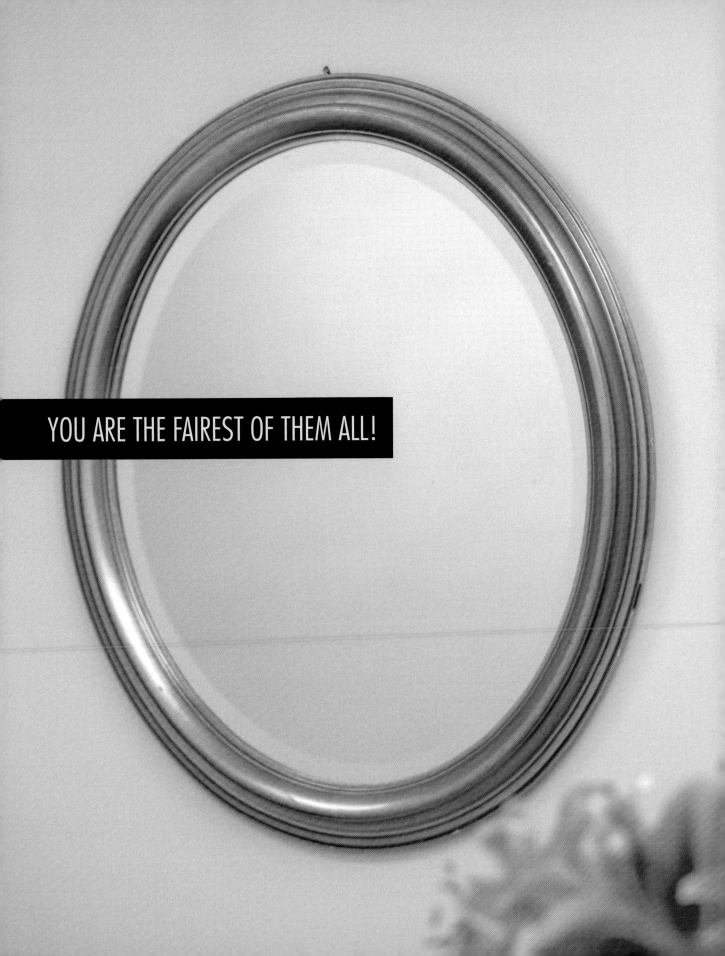

YOU ARE THE FAIREST OF THEM ALL!

NO TUGGING Close your eyes, take your hands, and run them over your face slowly. Allow your fingers to memorize the contours of your face. Pay attention to your cheekbones, the texture of your skin, the angles of your jaw. I know some of you are busy tugging at your loose chin, pulling back the skin on your cheeks and wondering about a face-lift. I promise we'll discuss plastic surgery later. For now, we're not concerned with fixing anything. Just like in a trial, during the initial period called "discovery" when the attorneys simply gather the facts of the case, discover your face with no criticisms or opinions. Remember, no tugging and no judging. Leave that to the plastic surgeons and the people in the black robes.

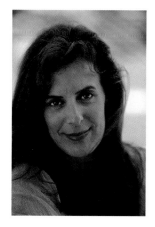

Now that you've investigated your face with your hands, open your eyes, brush your hair back away from your face, and look in the mirror. Focus on each feature separately: your hairline, your forehead, your brows, temples, eyes, eyelashes, nose, cheekbones, cheeks, lips, teeth, jawline, chin, and your complexion. Don't dwell on anything you consider negative, just study the quality of each unique feature.

Did it ever occur to you that somebody else's eyebrows simply wouldn't work on your face? How will you ever know what *will* work if you don't understand your unique attributes? Try answering these questions kindly, honestly, and with a degree of enthusiasm. If you lighten up on yourself, it can actually be fun.

KNOW THYSELF

- What is my favorite feature? Why?

- What feature do I receive the most compliments about?

- What color is my complexion? Light, medium, tan, or dark? What shade of foundation do I wear? Is the pigmentation on my face even?

- Does my skin burn easily in the sun?

- Do I have freckles? If so, do they contribute to my beauty?

- Do I like the way my eyebrows frame my face?

- What do my eyebrows suggest about my eyes?

- What do I like best about my eyes?

- Do they look happy or sad?

- What color are my eyes? How about the flecks inside my eyes?

- Are my eyes big or small in relationship to my face?

- How do my cheekbones define my face?

- Do I have a strong or weak jawline?

- Does my chin protrude?

- What shape is my nose? Is it wide or long?

- How would I describe the shape of my lips?

- Do I think I'm beautiful?

A helpful hint:

If you have trouble picking out your favorite feature, take a look at your makeup supplies. If you have a ton of lipsticks, chances are, you like your lips best. If you always get compliments on your eyes, you probably own a variety of shadows.

NOW YOU KNOW (AND YOU SURVIVED) Few of us take the time to look at ourselves intently and focus on the positive. This is because, believe it or not, most women rarely feel attractive. Did you think you were the only one? Even when you're told you look great, you really don't believe it, do you?

Though I've never seen you, if you're comparing yourself to a media icon, I know you're engaged in a losing battle. There's so much air-brushing and touching up of fashion photos, the models in real life don't even measure up to themselves. If you're comparing yourself to the way you looked twenty years ago, you won't get much out of that, either.

As women, we keep on getting better, so what's the point of getting stuck in a face from the past? Our possibilities are vast. It's time to get real, to see who you are right now, what you have, what you don't, and what you want to do about it.

REVEAL, DON'T MASK The self-evaluation should have helped you gain an objective understanding of how you look, a positive picture in your mind that will help you make smart decisions about your makeup. Now, let's move into the next portions of the book that will describe the various types of makeup and how to apply them. As you read, please feel free to take and leave what you like, according to what you just learned about your particular qualities. Once you know what you have to work with, you can accentuate and celebrate the beauty of your own face with makeup ideas.

These days, we no longer see tips in magazines like *Vogue* or *Harper's Bazaar* on how to contour your nose. Instead, we're learning to shift the focus of makeup from

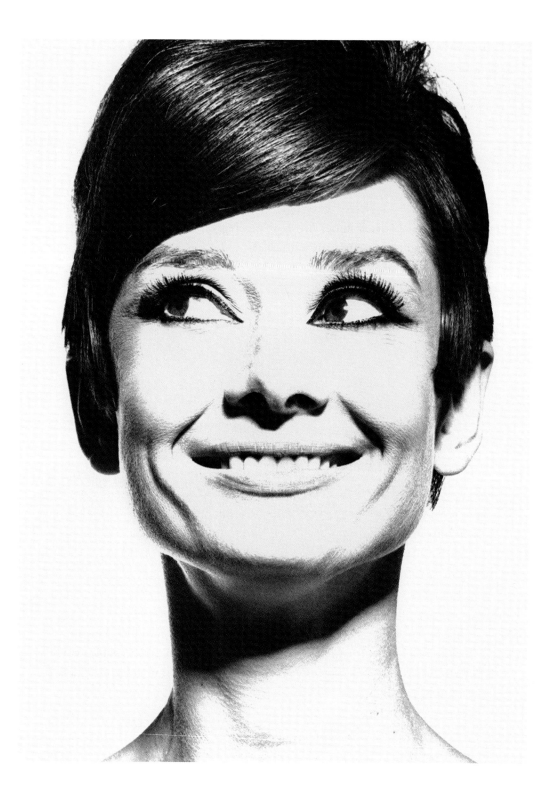

correcting to enhancing. I once worked with an actress who was accustomed to very unnatural contouring for her photo shoots. She expected me to draw heavy dark lines down the sides of her nose, but I had a different idea. I talked her out of unnatural shading on her nose by showing her how to make her eyes sparkle.

If you have dark circles under your eyes, covering them up with extremely light makeup really doesn't work. All you do is create raccoon eyes. Instead, use the techniques in the following pages to minimize the dark circles. Then, try drawing attention to your lips.

This is the beauty of doing a self-evaluation. You come away knowing what to highlight to make yourself shine. There's so much good about you. Be smart by learning to accept and accentuate your natural strengths. Once you've gained a positive picture of yourself, you can enhance your natural beauty with the power of makeup. Let's begin with the right tools.

MYTH:

IF YOU DON'T HAVE "PERFECT FEATURES," YOU'RE NOT BEAUTIFUL.

REALITY:

PERFECTION EXISTS IN HOW YOU FEEL ABOUT YOURSELF.

Uniqueness is finally being celebrated and appreciated, and not a moment too soon, I might add. In the old days, an oval face, a small, straight nose, almond-shaped eyes, impossibly high cheekbones, full lips, and a tiny waist were considered the criteria for beauty. Then along came Meryl Streep's very long nose, Anna Nicole Smith's full figure, Meg Ryan's thin lips, and Drew Barrymore's full cheeks. On their own, any of these features could be considered unattractive, but as a part of the whole, they contribute to the overall glamour of some exquisitely beautiful women.

The truth is that most of the women we think are classically beautiful have distinctive features that they themselves consider unattractive. Beauty is determined by a combination of your features, attitude, health, and elegance. When you get fixated on one of your features, you lose the perspective of seeing your face as the sum of its parts. If you want to look beautiful, don't change your nose. Change the way you feel about yourself.

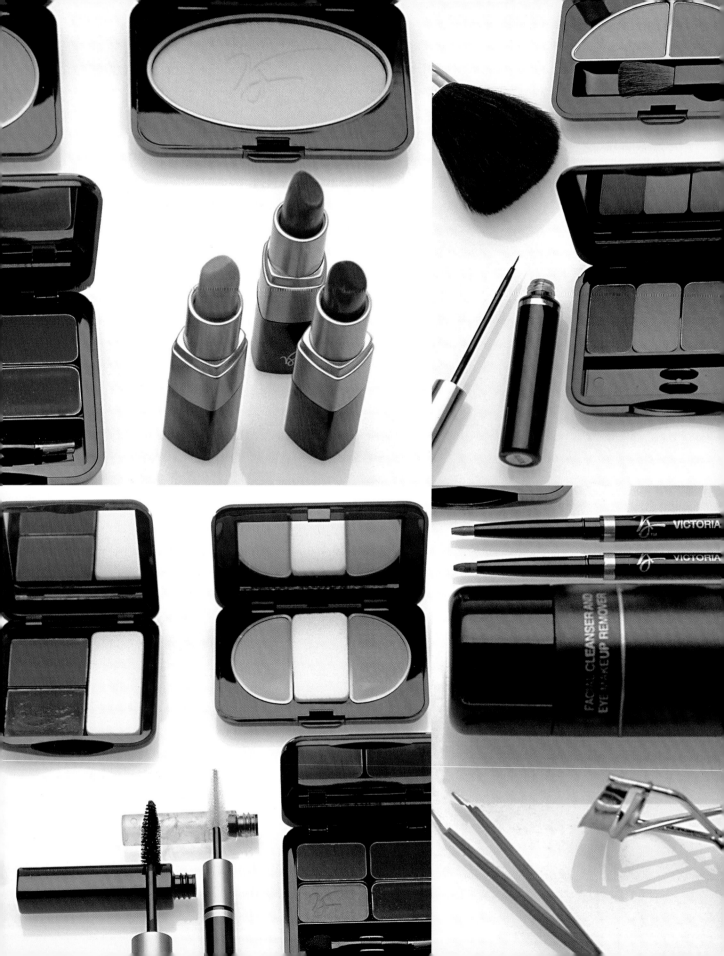

4: BUILDING YOUR BEAUTY ARSENAL

TAKING INVENTORY If you were to build a great wardrobe, you'd start by taking inventory and cleaning out the closet, getting rid of the outfits you haven't worn in a while because they're out of style, worn out, or they've never really looked good on you in the first place. I encourage you to approach building a working beauty arsenal in the same way. Go ahead, reach into the back of the drawers and pull out those old tubes of eyeliner and lipstick that have been taking up space and staining the wood on your dresser. It really is time to throw away that frothy-looking blue eye shadow that's not only out-of-date, but it's lost its consistency. You never found an appropriate place to wear it, anyway, so let it go. You wouldn't allow your wardrobe to be ten years behind the times, so why would you do that with your makeup collection?

Once you've cleared out what's old, take a look at what you have. It's time to take inventory, and the rewards are many. First, it always feels refreshing to get rid of old stuff to make room for the new. Secondly, you may find useful things you forgot you had. And finally, you probably own perfectly good items you've never used, simply because you didn't know what to do with them. Take heart—by the end of this chapter, you'll be rid of the things you don't want, you'll have a concise inventory of the tools you do have, you'll know what you need, and you'll have learned how and when to use them all.

FROM MASK TO ME Keep in mind that professional-looking results in makeup require tools that are clean, accessible, and in working order. There are so many wonderful products available today, designed to perform in a way that creates a natural look that is healthy for the skin.

In the past, we were less conscious than we are today about health, nutrition, and of course, makeup. We used makeup to create a mask, copying what we saw in magazines, sculpting and imitating looks that had nothing to do with us. Women wore heavier makeup on a daily basis, the consistencies were thicker, and the end results were unnatural. Eyes were lined to look like Cleopatra, blush was used to create sunken indentations in the cheeks, and eye shadows were so saturated with color, we couldn't find the eyes at all.

Trends have changed not only in the way we apply makeup, but the actual makeup itself. When you go out to replace some of the cosmetics as well as the tools in your arsenal, you'll find that everything has become much more refined. This may render your other products obsolete. I understand that spending money on a beauty arsenal can be a burden, but the better quality the tool, the better the results and the longer that tool will last. Sometimes, spending a little bit more on a better product proves more economical in the long run. I've taken a great deal of time over the years to compile the best available tools, and I manufactured some I couldn't find. I'll tell you what I use and then you can make decisions for yourself, based on finances and what you prefer. Remember—you don't have to do everything at once. Set your priorities and you can gradually fill in your beauty arsenal as you go along.

THE SPONGE Sponges are the number one item in my arsenal. A sponge is a forgiving beauty tool. It allows me control—to apply makeup easily, to blend off the edges, and to remove the excess. I package my foundation in a compact, in which I include a rectangular sponge that's great for touch-ups or applications on the run, but I use a latex wedge sponge whenever possible. In fact, I feel lost without one. The sharply defined edges of a wedge sponge make it easy to apply and smooth foundation in the small crevices around your nose and under your lower eyelashes. It also makes it easy to clean up excess base that often accumulates in laugh lines or other spots on your face.

The best way to choose the right sponge is to see what feels good on your face. Some sponges are irritating to the skin, and women can develop allergies to them, so this is a highly personal choice. I use high quality sponges, which I throw away after I've used all the sides once, not because I'm frivolous. I've just never found a way to clean them adequately, and they aren't expensive items. You can buy them in bulk in many pharmacies and beauty supply stores. If you can figure out how to clean them well enough, be my guest. If not, remember to use first one side, then the next, manipulating the wedge to get the most out of it before you retire it. The quality of your sponge will determine how much makeup it absorbs.

FOUNDATION, POWDER, AND BLUSH
Foundation is the first product I ever had manufactured, and it's one of the most popular products in my line. In the following chapters, I'll be going into foundation and the rest of the major makeup groups in detail, including when and how to use them and how to choose the best shades and types for you. For now, I'll say that I like a cream foundation, oil-free and sheer, for smoother application and the kind of coverage that allows the real skin to show through. I use my wedge sponge to apply it, and then I use the sponge once again to smooth and blend evenly.

After the foundation is lightly and evenly distributed, I use a neutral-toned translucent pressed powder. The purpose of powder is to absorb shine and any excess oils, not necessarily to deposit color. For a basic makeup application, a translucent powder will neutralize the foundation and remove the shine.

I apply powder with a compact-style puff, because it conforms so well to facial contours. I know that some women prefer a soft, thick brush. Whichever works best for you, the goal here is to choose a puff that absorbs the powder. If it sits on the puff, you end up with clumps of powder on your face. With a good puff, you won't get as much of what I call "pay-off," which means too much pigment deposited unequally. We're looking for less texture and more depth. Again, try out several types and decide for yourself. Just because I use something, doesn't mean it will work best for you.

To add color to the face, I use a powdered blush for the same reason I use a cream foundation—it allows me the best control. Cream blush is harder to apply and using it on uneven patches of skin, redness, or broken capillaries, can accentuate these problems and cause acne in some cases. I can achieve a natural kind of dusting with a blush powder, yet avoid changing the color too much. It also allows me to cover redness and achieve more of a natural glow.

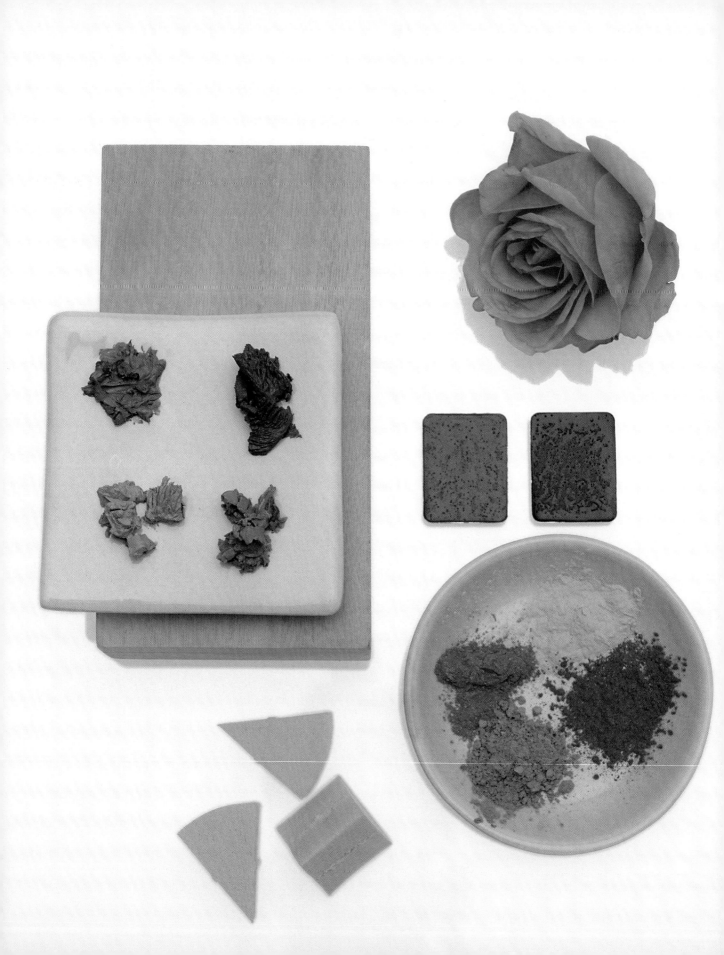

For blush application, I use a big, fluffy brush, about one-half inch at its bristle base. This type feels good on my face and helps deposit color in a natural way. Once you get used to a blush brush with a long handle, chances are the compact size will no longer please you. I suggest a retractable brush (it fits in your purse) that offers length and soft full bristles.

A final word on brushes: Just as a bad sponge can irritate your skin and cause break-outs, so can a bad brush. A good brush will last a long time, a year or two, depending on how you care for it. So here again, spending a little bit more will usually benefit you in longevity and usefulness. If you want your brush to last, clean it regularly and watch the stress you're putting on it.

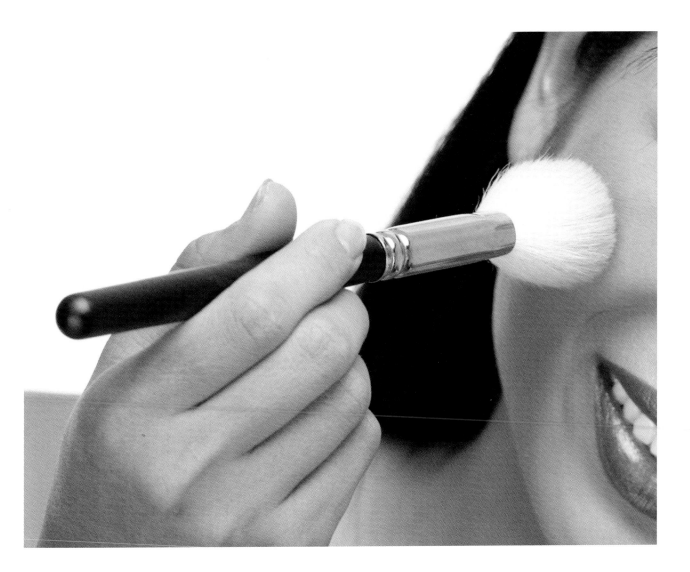

THE EYES: BROWS, LASHES, LINER, AND SHADOW
In order to keep your eyebrows well-groomed, a good tweezer is an important tool. I like the Tweezerman brand, since it allows me to firmly grasp the hair and to effect a quick, thorough removal. Whether you choose a tweezer with a slanted tip or a pointy tip is personal preference, so be sure to test them out for yourself. After tweezing, I use a brow brush to keep the brows even.

In my line of cosmetics, I have a wonderful taupe eyebrow pencil that I suggest for the majority of women. Its very soft lead helps define the brows in a hair-like way, and it works for light, medium, and dark complexions. Women of color will probably want to use a dark brown pencil which I also manufacture, but I don't suggest black for most people. Even though we've seen exotic beauties with naturally black eyebrows, for most women, it's a little too harsh.

For applying eyeliner, I use a brown or black pencil. Again, a soft lead allows you to smudge easily and to get right down into the lash line. Since you're working so close to the eye, you need to find a pencil that doesn't irritate you. By the way, I keep the edges of my pencil rounded, not sharp, to create a softer, more natural look. I sharpen it and press the tip down on the palm of my hand to round it out.

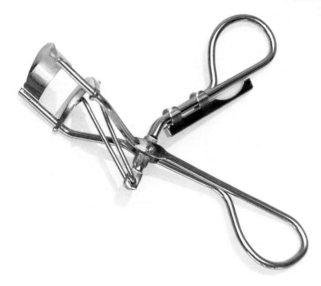

Makeup shouldn't have sharp points, so I don't like tools with sharp points, either. Though I don't have liquid eyeliner in my line, I use it on rare occasions to create a little more intensity. Feel free to experiment. Just make sure you apply the liquid with a really fine brush to create depth without creating an unnaturally thick line. Go slowly with liquid, because once applied, it's harder to blend than pencil.

Before applying mascara, I use an eyelash curler. I find that curling your lashes helps open the eyes and adds length to the lashes. Once the lashes are curled and lengthened, I use my duo mascara with sheer on one side, which I highly recommend for teens, and brown or black on the other. For adults, using the sheer side first creates a nice base on which to add color.

Whichever brand of mascara you decide to use, make sure the brush builds and separates the lashes, and the formula isn't too wet or too dry. Wide spaces between bristles will allow for clumps, so check the brush carefully. After applying the mascara, I use the comb side of my brow brush to separate the lashes and to avoid clumps. The more you pump the wand into the tube, the more air gets into it, and that can draw bacteria. I only recommend a waterproof mascara when necessary for swimming, beach days, and emotional times. The downside of waterproof mascara is that you have to work a little harder to remove it, sometimes irritating your eyes and possibly losing precious eyelashes.

A nice subtle eye shadow completes the eyes. Both creams and powder eye shadows are available, but I prefer powders for easiest application. I tend to go light on the shadow, using it mainly to define and accentuate. I like to use a professional brush with a slant tip for defining and uplifting the eye. I use the rounder side for filling in color. The spongy type brushes are good for touch-ups, but, in general, I prefer hair brushes.

LIPS

I want to let you in on a Hollywood secret. To cover fine lines around lips, dip the tip of your lip brush into my cream foundation, and line your lips before applying lipstick. If you like to use lip liner to stop lipstick from bleeding into fine lines, do it with a lip pencil. I like a very fine, retractable one that fits easily in my purse. On a general basis, though, women are using colored lip liner a lot less these days.

My lip compacts have four shades in them. I enjoy mixing colors even for touch-ups, and a good lip brush makes it that much easier. I put my lip creams in a compact because I don't like tubes clanking around and getting lost in my purse. I like the texture of cream, it's easy to apply with a lip brush, and I enjoy having extra choices as the day goes on.

MAKEUP REMOVER

It's always important to have a good eye makeup remover to correct any mishaps during your application. I use it faithfully every night to remove all my makeup. You should go to bed with a clean face, to keep your skin healthy and looking its best. There are many different formulas on the market, from the old-fashioned standards like Pond's cold cream and Vaseline, to some newer improved versions like creams, pads, gels, or lotions. I love my remover, because it has the consistency of water and doesn't leave any residue. I'm also partial to it for its dual purposes. It removes makeup and corrects mistakes and it was also formulated to be used as a facial cleanser.

EXTRAS

To fill out your beauty arsenal, it's good to have some cotton swabs, Q-tips, and Kleenex on hand, for blending and correcting. Although I don't use them frequently, oil-control blotting papers can be handy in a pinch to reduce oil on your face.

YOUR FUN BASKET

Every woman should have her fun basket with false eyelashes as well as the exotic eye shadow and lipstick colors you wouldn't wear to the office or the supermarket. For you confirmed party girls, try playing with the new wildly colored mascaras. All glittery and shiny makeup items belong in this basket. Think *Viva Las Vegas*!

BEING FOREARMED IS A GOOD THING

Evaluating your beauty arsenal is in essence, an extension of evaluating your face. Once you find out what you have and what you don't, and then learn how to use it, you can do a realistic make-over that helps you feel better about yourself.

You don't need to rush out and get everything at once. Buy what you need immediately and slowly expand until you have everything you need to feel secure and to be able to do your makeup quickly and effectively. When you have the right tools in working order, it gives you an added edge. A head start. Being forearmed for the best makeup job is another good way to put makeup behind you. Then you can move out into the world with enough self-assurance to get on with the rest of your life.

HELPFUL HINTS:

- If you develop a rash or an allergy on your face, it may be the sponge, not the makeup. Try a different sponge before you change your makeup product.

- Buy brushes according to how they feel on your face. If they're scratchy or have hairs falling out, they won't be effective or long-lasting.

- Black eyebrows are unnatural-looking on most women.

- Keep the edges of your eyeliner pencil rounded, not sharp, to create a softer, more natural look by pressing the tip into the palm of your hand.

- Don't keep a mascara wand longer than three months, as it tends to dry out and attract bacteria.

BEAUTY MARK
1:
Working with sponges will make a huge difference in your overall beauty application. Fingers work, but sponges are better.

BEAUTY MARK
2:
An investment in a set of good brushes will pay off in the end.

BEAUTY MARK
3:
To cover fine lines around lips, dip the tip of your lip brush into cream foundation, and line your lips before applying lipstick.

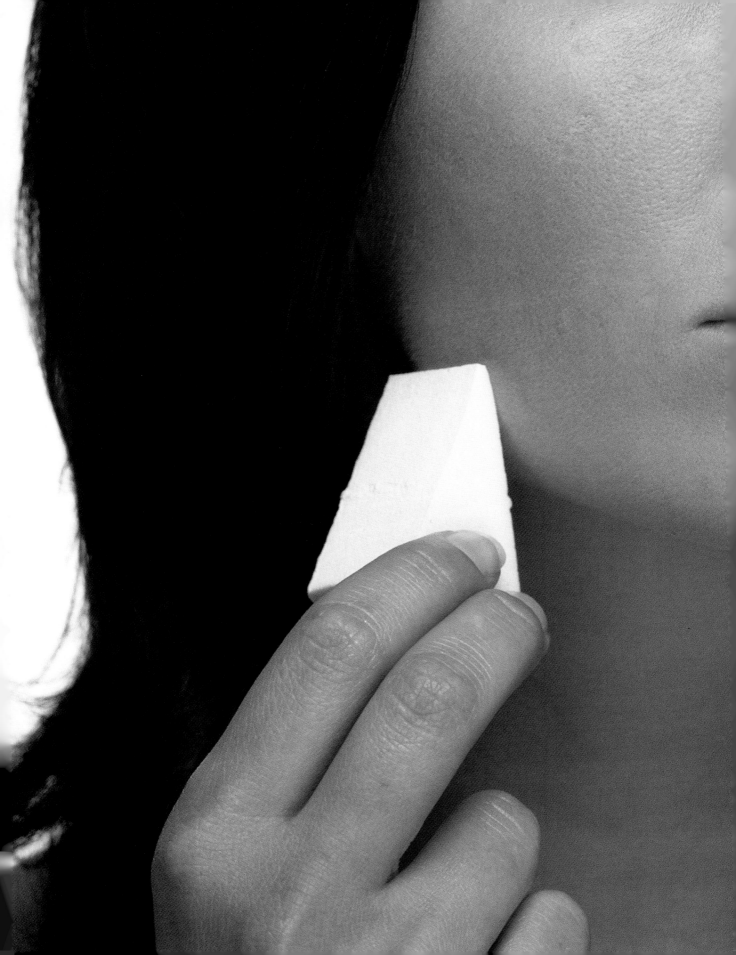

5: FOUNDATION & POWDER: WHERE IT ALL BEGINS

FABULOUS FOUNDATION It's fitting that foundation was the first product I created. When we work on the foundation of who we are and how we view things, it feels as if we're smoothing out the lines of life and becoming more at peace with ourselves. I like to think of foundation as character, the bottom line upon which everything else gets built.

A weak foundation in life ultimately creates a poor result, just as building a color palette on the wrong shade or texture of foundation won't work. A good foundation offers you a solid base, an opportunity to look beyond your flaws and imperfections and to focus on what's right instead of what's wrong. If you have a sense of security, intelligence, knowledge, and a comfort level at your base, everything you build on top of that will be strong and secure. Have you ever noticed that if you spend all your time thinking about what's wrong with you, that's what you'll reflect to the outside world? In the same way, when you apply your makeup on a base that you don't feel good about, your look will fall apart. It's like trying to build a dream house from the top down.

If you think of your face as a blank canvas with the foundation setting the background, then you can create a flawless, even texture over which color, shadow, and highlights can be laid. Once you've covered distractions like spots, under-eye circles, redness, spider veins, or broken capillaries, applying the rest of your makeup becomes that much easier because you can envision the future possibilities. "I have beautiful eyes," you might say, "but they weren't visible before when all I could see was my acne."

A good foundation can create a flawless, even canvas, helping you broaden your view of yourself.

SHEER IS HERE! I created my foundation (incidentally, the most popular product in my line) not so much as a fulfillment of a dream, but as an antidote to frustration. Clear, even-toned skin is a major component of beauty, and, being a perfectionist, I was unhappy with the quality of available foundations, both in color and texture. For starters, they all contained the most unnatural shades of oranges and pinks, which don't blend properly with anybody's skin.

As hard as I searched, I could find nothing with a yellow base, which is a far more natural skin tone color. In fact, from ivory to the darkest foundation shades, a yellow undertone is crucial to your foundation appearing and feeling like a second skin. To add to the problem, the products on the market at that time were much too thick, resulting in a pasty, made-up look. This did not fit into my "no makeup makeup" philosophy. Something new was definitely needed.

I envisioned a foundation that would be effective enough in consistency to cover flaws such as blemishes, dark spots, scarring or undereye dark circles. At the same time, it had to be sheer enough to allow the real skin to shine through. I knew what I wanted, but how could I, a woman with little money and no experience in cosmetic chemistry, create a brand-new concept in makeup?

Undaunted by my lack of resources, motivated by a great desire to have what I envisioned, I started mixing up my own concoctions in pots and pans in my garage. I found several different foundations that had some sense of the shades I wanted, and when I reached an impasse, I took my concept to a chemist. I didn't realize at the time that I'd chosen one of the biggest and best cosmetic chemists in the country.

"I have this idea," I told him, speaking quickly so he wouldn't dismiss me. "It's something brand-new—natural foundation shades, more yellow-based, that'll make a woman's skin look perfect. I'm a Hollywood makeup artist and I don't have any money, but I know it can work. Please, will you help? I promise to give you all my future purchase orders."

I was offering him first dibs on nothing right then, but as luck would have it, this wonderful man agreed to work with me. Why he did it still boggles my mind. It might have been that I was so persistent, he just didn't have the heart to refuse me. Maybe my enthusiasm was contagious, maybe he liked the challenge of doing something new, or maybe he saw the wisdom in my idea. Whatever the reason, it paid off for both of us. Years later, when I was in a position to go into mass manufacturing, this man became my biggest manufacturer, and as I write this, he still is.

THE FOUR-STEP APPLICATION IN LESS THAN A MINUTE
Many women prefer not to use foundation all over their faces, but to spot it here and there. I'm all for that. If you're basically happy with the texture of your skin but you need to cover a blemish or some other imperfection, pick up a tiny drop of foundation on your sponge and dab it on the problem area. Sometimes that's all it takes. For larger blemishes or scarring, or for complete coverage for any reason, follow my four application steps.

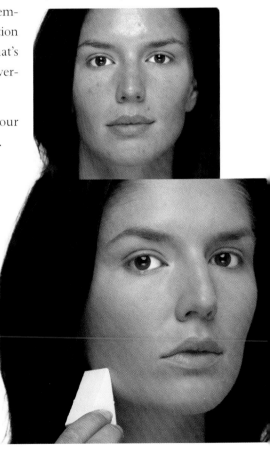

1   Dab your sponge into the foundation and apply to your jawline in a smooth, downward stroke toward the chin.

2   Once you've covered the jaw, under the jaw, and the chin, make downward strokes with the sponge all over your face. Remember to blend carefully under your lashes, around your nose and brows, and into the hairline. Blend, blend, blend.

3   For dark areas under the eyes or around the nose, use foundation that is one-half to one shade lighter than the base. Paint the shadows with a brush and blend lightly with a sponge.

4   Finally, lightly apply translucent powder over your entire face. Be sure to distribute it evenly. Areas that need special attention are the forehead, nose, and chin where oils tend to accumulate.

39

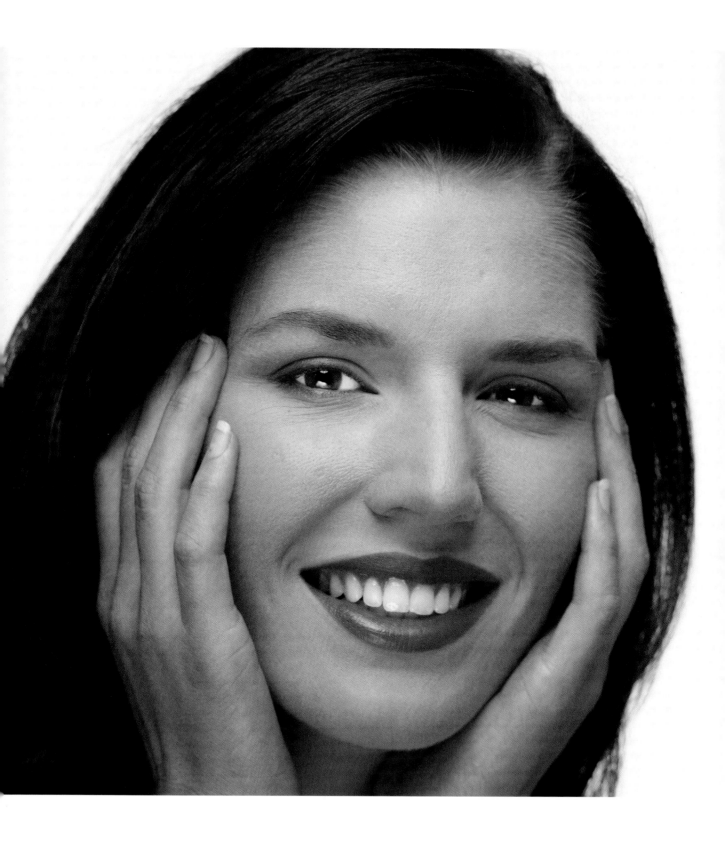

Remember to apply foundation in downward strokes so the natural peach fuzz we all have stays smooth and unnoticeable. Before powdering, dab extra foundation on problem areas, blend again, go back with a powder puff and apply powder to the problem areas once again. That should do it!

The bottom line on foundation is that less is more. Who wants to look like she's wearing gunk on her face? A small amount of foundation applied evenly creates a natural sheen and a flawless finish. Skin imperfections can be easily covered up with a light application of the right shade, and the new, sheer foundations are lightweight and a pleasure to wear. Once you've perfected use of the sponge, it should take less than a minute to apply your foundation.

Makeup that is poorly blended is easy to correct. Simply take a wedge sponge and smooth it gently over your skin to remove excess makeup and to blend the shade until your skin tone looks even.

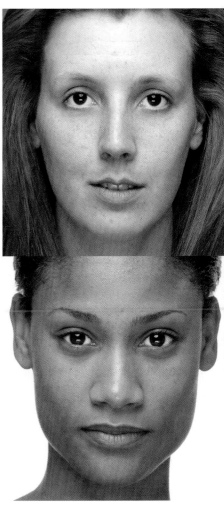

GUIDELINES FOR
LIGHTER SKIN TONES:

- Skin tends to take on more color in summer whether you protect it or not. Have a second foundation shade available, just in case.

- Pink-toned foundations are always a no-no.

- If your neck is noticeably lighter than your face, even out the contrast with a slightly deeper foundation shade and blend into your neck well.

GUIDELINES FOR
DARKER SKIN TONES:

- Avoid talc or titanium ingredients, as they give an ashy appearance to the skin.

- Bring up darker areas with a lighter shade. Leave a little variation in tone which looks natural.

- Choose a mid-tone foundation between the darker areas and the lighter ones. Some companies will custom-blend a foundation shade, but remember that the shade is only as good as the makeup artist who does the blending.

41

THE TWO C'S: CONCEAL AND CAMOUFLAGE

As a makeup artist, I found the thing that causes women the most concern is concealing—everything from under-eye dark circles to acne, from skin discolorations to broken capillaries. The biggest mistake women make is using either a foundation shade or a concealer that's too light. This will draw more attention to the trouble area, and will not help you achieve the corrective results.

I've found that with the right foundation, you may not need concealer at all. At certain times, though, a concealer may give you the extra coverage you need to even out skin tones and cover dark circles. Concealers come in liquid, cream, or stick. With my foundation, all you need to do is use a half-shade lighter than the under-eye dark circles. If the foundation doesn't do the trick, try a cream concealer which I think is the easiest to apply. Keep in mind that yellow and neutral beige undertones are foolproof for most skins.

Remember—don't make the mistake of trying to hide dark circles with a shade so light, it creates a white mask around your eyes. I call that creating "reverse raccoon eyes." It only accentuates and draws attention to a problem. Blue under-eye circles, often found on people with deep-set eyes, are generally caused by veins that are visible through this very thin skin. Use eye cream to smooth out skin texture, and then concealer, taking care with that delicate skin.

If you have a hyper-pigmentation problem like large brown spots or deep scarring, pancake or stick makeup might be the best choice. Only in extreme cases do I resort to bringing in the heavy artillery to cover a significant flaw, a process I call camouflaging. I prefer to conceal, which makes a subtle difference with a light application of foundation.

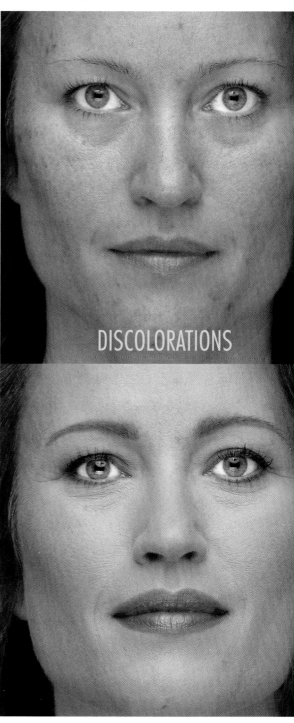

DISCOLORATIONS

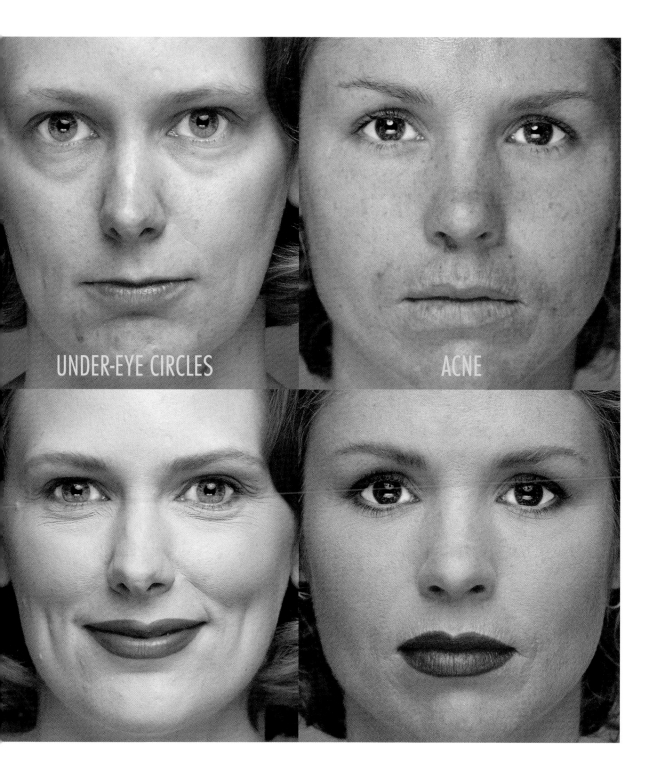

UNDER-EYE CIRCLES

ACNE

MAKING THE RIGHT CHOICE I always advise women that they don't *have* to wear foundation, and I mean it. Some women look wonderful and feel more comfortable without a base, but I'm here to tell you that no one has "perfect" skin. The flawless faces you see in the movies and in fashion magazines are achieved by using a foundation that refines the look of a woman's complexion. She may look as if she has nothing on her skin, but believe me, a good foundation is what you're not seeing.

Selecting the right foundation is crucial to the "no makeup makeup" look. There are many different choices in the marketplace from creams to sticks, from liquids to powders, and it's fine to use whatever you like best. But first you need to determine if your skin is dry, oily, a combination of the two, or very, very sensitive. It's always good to stick with allergy-tested cosmetics, and know which chemicals, if any, irritate your particular skin. This may take some experimentation, but it'll be worth it in the long run.

Most doctors agree that alcohol, SD alcohol, fragrances, glycols, lanolin, mineral oils, petrolatum, and preservatives tend to cause allergic reactions for sensitive skin, so check the ingredients in your makeup before you buy it.

To help you make the right choice, here's a breakdown of the many types available:

- WATER-BASED LIQUID: This is good for people who are more acne-prone and have lots of natural oils in their skin. But be careful. Just because it's called water-based doesn't mean it has no oil. It just may have more water than oil. My experience is that this type doesn't give the most even coverage.

- OIL-FREE LIQUID: If your skin is very sensitive and you break out easily, try this as a solution. The only trouble here is that without any oil at all, a liquid foundation may streak or appear chalky on application.

- POWDER-FORMULATED FOUNDATION: This type of foundation will create a finished, natural look. It works well for normal to oily skin.

- TINTED MOISTURIZER: This provides threefold benefits: It evens out the skin, moisturizes, and provides skin protection. It often contains oil, so check the labels and take it easy at first to see what happens.

- CREAM: My personal favorite, a cream foundation brings radiance to the skin. My formula is non-oily and with a little powder to absorb shine, I think it gives the best coverage.

- PANCAKE OR STICK: Definitely the heaviest coverage. I suggest this only for people who need to camouflage.

Foundations to avoid:

- MULTIPHASE FOUNDATION: This requires mixing because the alcohol or water settles on the top, while talc and pigment fall to the bottom. It ends up dry and chalky on the skin, and is only recommended for severe cases of acne.

- LONG-WEARING SMUDGE-PROOF FOUNDATION: Unnatural foundation that doesn't blend and is harsh to the skin. Any amount of money spent here is wasted.

- TWO-IN-ONE FORMULAS: Whether it's cream and then powder or liquid and powder, it steals your control over the final effect.

- WET/DRY FORMULAS: This looks floury on the skin in dry form, while the wet form ends up looking thick.

Many of the newest foundations can do two or even three jobs in one. Check the ingredients for these valuable extras:

- SPF: If you live in a year-round sunny climate, this is very important. Many tinted moisturizers and liquid foundations come with built in sunscreen, as does my cream formula.

- AHA/BHA: The concentration of alpha- and beta-hydroxy acids is far less than the amount found in designated skin care products, but they do have a mild exfoliant effect. Overuse can irritate skin, so avoid the eye area if these ingredients are included.

- ANTIOXIDANTS: A, C, and E are the vitamins most used here to place free-radical fighters at the surface of the skin. Sensitive skin could break out so test on a small area first.

- OIL ABSORBERS: Kaolin and talc absorb excess facial oil and give the skin a matte appearance. Be careful they don't settle into fine lines.

- MOISTURIZERS: Emollients, generally some type of oil, provide a lightweight barrier that keeps moisture from evaporating. Allows the skin to feel less taut and more comfortable.

Keep the weather in mind when you're choosing foundation or any other makeup. Your skin texture changes in the summer and winter, so be sure to give your skin what it needs.

Let me remind you that whether you use my line or any other, what's important is that you find a foundation with a shade and a texture that feels light and looks invisible. It should almost feel like a second skin. When you're choosing color, think shade, texture, and intensity. When my clients find a shade and consistency that best suits their complexion and their expectations, I suggest they don't stray from it. Actually, one shade is what you need most of the time, because if you're committed to soft, beautiful, healthy skin, you won't be out there getting a tan on your face. For those who insist on catching a few rays or find themselves in the garden without a hat, I suggest you select a foundation one-half to one shade darker than you use on the rest of your face. And always use some form of sunscreen to combat the carcinogenic effects of the sun. Nothing ages a woman faster than burning the sensitive skin on her face.

In choosing your perfect color foundation, you can safely eliminate bases with gray, pink, or orange undertones. These are simply not natural skin tones. If your skin has excess redness, yellow or neutral undertones in a base will help to cut through it, while pinks and oranges will create a muddy, artificial look.

It's important that the shade you use matches both your face and your neck, so testing makeup on your wrist doesn't make sense. Use the area of your jawbone, instead. I can't say it enough that makeup is all about applying, layering, and blending, one thing building naturally upon the next. If you create a line of demarcation with your neck a darker shade than your face or vice versa, it'll look like you're wearing a mask.

POWDER PERFECT After applying foundation, I like to use powder to create a more matte look, reducing the shine and absorbing oils. It also acts as a protective layer, holding the foundation in place on your skin. Oil-controlled powders will help you touch up what I call "break-out shine" throughout the day.

Powder is available in different forms: loose or pressed. I prefer pressed because I like to work with a puff that will give me a more controlled application. The puff will absorb excess

For me, beauty is much more than how you look from a cosmetic point of view. Great skin, shiny hair, and good bones all help. But as I get older, I know that it's what's inside, shining through.

— Ali MacGraw

Dear Victoria,

My skin is uneven and pale, and when I use a good foundation, I feel confident that I look pretty and that it won't irritate my skin. Before I learned how to blend it, I always had a line by my chin area so you could tell I was wearing foundation. As you know, that's not the case any more. I also used to need cover up, (a stick) for under my eyes, but the foundation takes care of everything.

—C. L. West Bend, IA

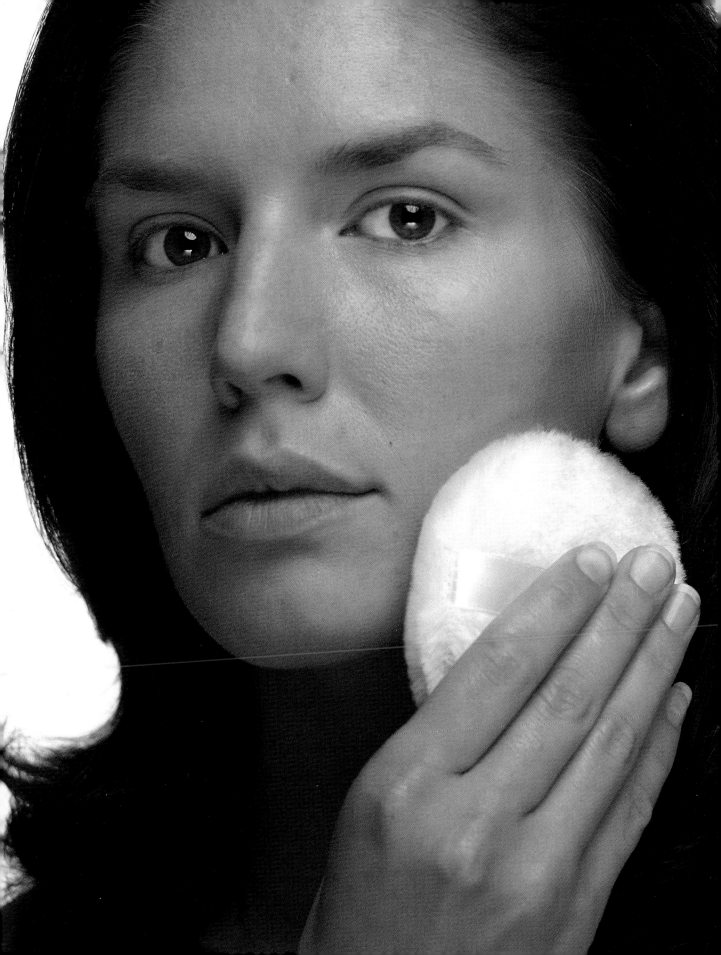

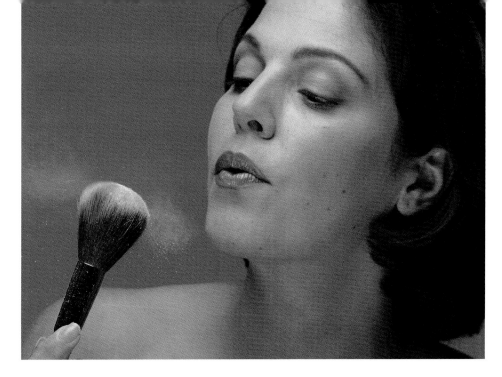

powder, allowing me to leave the right amount on my face. Key to remember about powder—you're not using it solely to add color. Let your blush and shadows be the color sources. Powder is mainly for reducing shine and should feel light as air and silky in your hand.

By the way, too little powder leaves an oilier look while too much will leave your foundation looking heavy or cakey. The surest way to create a heavy look is to cover your foundation with a ton of powder. The powder will accumulate in the fine lines of your skin, drawing attention to wrinkles.

If you like to wear powder without foundation underneath it, test the powder on your bare skin to achieve the desired result. If you wear it over foundation, make sure you are using your customary shade of foundation when you choose a powder for your face. There are powder blotting papers available in drugstores that are economical, easy to carry, and will help reduce shine on the face throughout the day.

HELPFUL HINTS:

- Your jawline is the best area on which to test foundation. When a stroke of your base is invisible, that's a perfect match.

- Indoor lighting can create illusions, so match colors in natural lighting.

- For under-eye dark circles, use a foundation one-half tone lighter than the shade of the dark circles. Be careful with concealers which are often too thick to conceal.

- Don't try to hide under-eye circles with light makeup. That's what creates raccoon eyes.

- If you decide to tan lightly in the summer, choose a foundation one-half to one shade darker than your normal shade.

- Don't try altering your skin shade with foundation. Instead, choose a shade that closely matches your own complexion color.

- To make touch-ups easier, keep a few oil-control blotting papers in your purse to reduce that oily look.

- Use a translucent powder to absorb oil and avoid extra color.

- Too much powder under the eyes can crack and crumble, producing that cakey, aging effect.

- When dipping brush into loose powder, blow it off the brush to avoid caking it on face.

- Contouring a wide nose with dark foundation is unnatural and only draws attention to it. Instead of trying to correct a problem, remove the focus by accentuating one of your favorite features.

BEAUTY MARK

1:

Less is more.

BEAUTY MARK

2:

Choose a shade most natural to your skin tone, and apply sparingly.

BEAUTY MARK

3:

Envision this first step as the beginning of infinite possibilities.

APPLICATIONS for FOUNDATION

MINIMAL TO LIGHT FOUNDATION

Most women only need a light application of foundation. Always remember—less is best. Use minimal foundation when it is only needed and desired in specific areas to cover a mole, broken capillaries, or one or more blemishes.

- Foundation creates a smooth, flawless base so you can accent your best features!

- When mixing two shades, dab sponge lightly in each, concentrating more on whichever color matches your neck color. Only a small amount is needed.

- Apply foundation in downward motion to minimize impact of facial hair.

- Foundation should be applied very lightly so that your skin is visible underneath. It is prettiest when blended into your skin, not sitting on top.

- Dab sponge on problem areas only.

- If desired, cover entire face in downward motion.

- Blend color on face. Make sure to blend around and under jawline, into hairline, on earlobes if they are a different color, around nose, around eye up to the bottom lash line, and under brow.

- Dab one area of face as need for extra coverage.

- Lightly powder to set foundation.

A HEAVY FOUNDATION

To cover acne, problem skin, or cover freckles completely.

- Apply foundation on face so no skin is visible through foundation.

- If one area needs more concentration of coverage, apply with a dabbing touch, called "stippling."

- Lightly powder to set foundation.

- Concentrate heaviest application by stippling puff on problem areas.

- You can also cover freckles and birthmarks in this manner. Make sure to match your shade to the skin on that particular area. Do not try to lighten only the area in which you are working, or you will draw more attention to the problem.

DARK CIRCLES UNDER EYES

- Apply lightest shade foundation with a wedged sponge.

- Only go one-half to one shade lighter than the under-eye dark area.

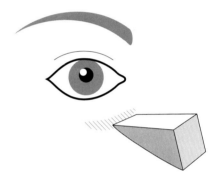

- Using too light of a shade will result in a "Raccoon Eye Effect," which makes the circles look worse.

1 Place lighter color under eye in the dark circle.

2 Blend with foundation sponge.

3 If more coverage is desired, add more color in circle with brush and blend with sponge.

4 Lightly powder to set.

UNDER-EYE BAGS AND PUFFINESS

- With wedged sponge, dip into lightest shade of foundation.

- Always use mirror for placement of lighter color in bag or puffy area.

1 Add lighter foundation in shadow/bag. You will notice a slight shadow on sides of puffiness. Add lighter color there, also.

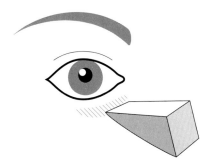

2 Blend softly.

3 Do not add light color on top of puffiness. You want to shade the puffiness to recess and highlight the bag/shadow to bring up.

4 For shading puffiness, using darker foundation color, carefully dab puffiness only, with tip of wedged sponge or cotton swab. Be light-handed.

5 Blend lightly with sponge.

6 Lightly powder to set foundation.

MINIMIZING FACIAL LINES AROUND NOSE AND MOUTH

1 Dip tip of wedged sponge into lightest foundation color.

2 Apply lighter color in deepest area of line.

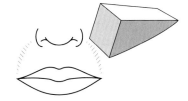

3 Blend lightly up to highest point outside of line with sponge.

4 Powder lightly to set foundation.

5 Don't go more than one-half shade to one shade lighter or you will draw attention to the problem.

TO EMPHASIZE CHEEKBONES

- Suck in cheeks and using fingertips, softly press under cheekbones until you feel hollow. Press along hollow from ear to cheek, stopping before center, aligning with eyes. This is the area to be contoured, following the natural bone structure you feel.

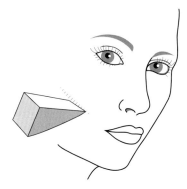

1 With wedge sponge or cotton swab, use foundation to draw line in hollow under cheekbone, from ear to center, aligning with eye.

2 Lightly blend down cheek and blend into cheekbone to soften. Darkest concentration will be in hollow.

3 Do not blend too high on cheekbone. This is your natural highlight. Blend to a gentle shading.

4 Lightly powder to set foundation.

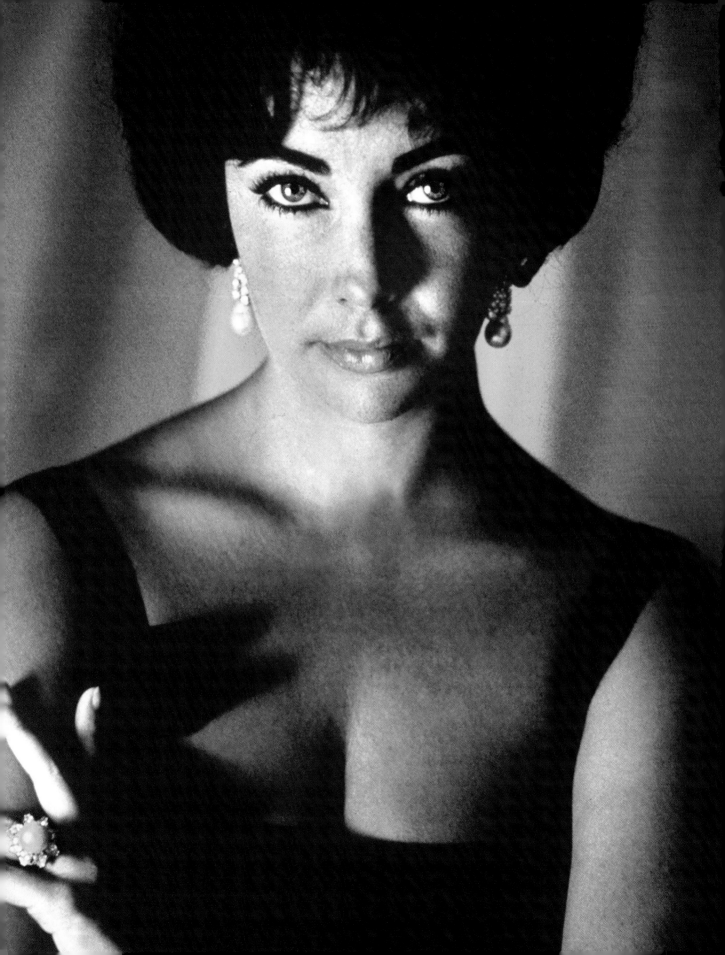

6: EYEBROWS: THE FACE'S EXCLAMATION POINTS

SIGN OF THE TIMES Eyebrows tend to be the most neglected part of a woman's makeup. For some reason, women tend to pay more attention to their eyeliner and shadow. This may be because up close in the mirror, it's difficult to see how the brows frame the face. When you step back and view the big picture, you'll see how the eyebrows frame the eyes, giving the entire face life, strength, and expression. They can open the face, lift deep-set eyes, or make small ones appear larger. When a woman's eyelids tend to sag as she gets older, creating the right shape brows will open the eyes. Brows shaped and colored correctly are a natural disguise and can take years off!

I see the brows as the face's exclamation points, accentuating the eyes' most subtle and dramatic forms of communication. When a woman wants to make exciting changes in her makeup, I always look to the eyebrows to begin that process.

Since brow styles shift decidedly with the times, shaping the eyebrows is a definitive way to keep up with fashion trends. For a quick review, let's go back to the fifties, when Marilyn Monroe and Elizabeth Taylor wore their eyebrows full at the base, tapering off to near nothingness as they reached the temples. Brows began to fill out in the next decade, transforming the sophisticated, alluring look of the previous beauty queens to that of a more innocent, natural brow. Audrey Hepburn and Twiggy are two distinctly different examples of stunning women with sixties-style brows, a natural beauty shining through each of their individual and powerful senses of personal style.

Women headed for the workplace *en masse* in the seventies, creating a dramatic shift, where a perfectly groomed brow became the most popular makeup statement. By the eighties, women were a permanent fixture in the workforce, having assumed a certain degree of power over their own lives. Brooke Shields's furry eyebrows, accenting her all-around vitality as well as her gorgeous eyes, demonstrated women's newfound sense of themselves.

The nineties were all about reaching a balance, where brows returned to gentle contouring with soft arches. Without giving up the power and self-confidence which we had clearly established for ourselves, women wanted to accentuate a more refined and feminine quality of life. Today, we have brought with us all that went before. Women can look beautiful with almost any style of brow they choose, as long as it is nicely groomed. I prefer a brow that's left a bit fuller in the center with a soft peak, the rest of the brow trailing out to the end and moving in a subtle upward direction. "Natural" is the overwhelming style in the new millennium as women stand straight, strong, and feminine, proud of who we have become.

REFRAMING YOUR ATTITUDE When you're about to make up your eyebrows, think of yourself as a framer, trying to bring out the best in a wonderful painting—your face. Once you've covered your canvas with a flawless, even background (the foundation), ask yourself which frame will make your face come alive. Would you take a beautiful painting filled with light and

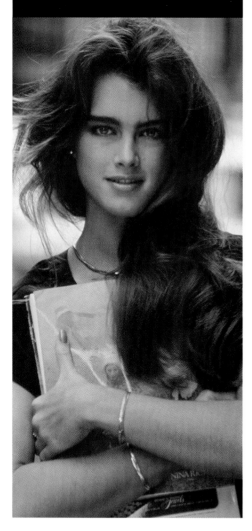

"Beauty is an attitude. If you feel good about yourself, you shine as a person. That, to me, is beauty."
— *Ole Henriksen,*
skin care expert

color, and stick a dark, pointy, oddly shaped frame around it? Of course not. An overpowering frame that calls attention to itself will detract from the canvas, minimizing the impact of the painting.

I've seen dramatic demonstrations of the way the brows frame the face and determine a woman's attitude at Sybil Brand Institute, a maximum security county jail for women in Los Angeles. With the help of my sister Audrey, who's in charge of the LA County Sheriff's Psychological Department, I implemented a self-esteem program for women who were about to be released from jail. My idea was to design a makeup class to help them feel more secure about fitting in when they first ventured out into the world. They responded positively. Even the female guards stood around and listened, proving once again that women everywhere in nearly all professions love makeup.

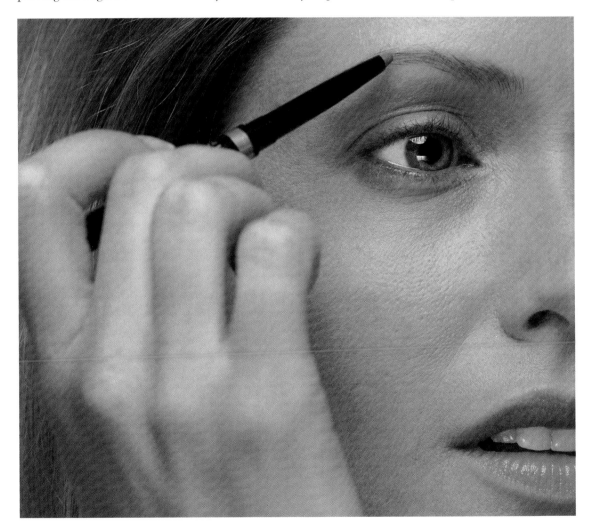

I began the class by asking the women to consider the message they wanted their makeup to suggest.

"Pull over," one of the women answered.

I laughed good-naturedly at her comment and then I answered her obvious challenge. "What if your makeup said, 'Stop and look at me. I care about myself. I'm important, and I have respect for myself.'"

As we continued to talk, I noticed that in prison, eyebrows spoke loudly and carried major attitude. Some of the women, rather than tweezing their eyebrows, were in the habit of shaving them off completely. Others shaved them partly off, using a razor to shape what was left into pointy, mean-looking peaks above the center of their eyes. If their intention was to look ganglike, scary, and unapproachable, they had certainly achieved their goal. This message would do nothing positive for them in the outside world, so I wanted to show them how they might approach their makeup differently.

I asked how many of the hundred or so women attending my workshop were shaving their eyebrows. A good number of hands went up. I picked one of the women, (she was about twenty), with what I call "angry eyebrows," and asked her if I could use her for an experiment. When she agreed, I took my taupe eyebrow pencil and softened the arch of one of her eyebrows, lightly penciling in what she had shaved off. I left the other eyebrow as it was. Then I asked the entire group of women to vote on which look they preferred. I knew I'd get an honest show of hands, as these women were not prone to telling lies to make somebody else feel good.

The vote was unanimous. They all preferred the softer look. When I offered the young woman a mirror, she agreed the arch looked too hard and she wanted me to show her what I'd done so she could make the other eyebrow match. Right before my eyes, a visible shift occurred in her attitude. What a rewarding moment it was for me as I watched her become a little bit more comfortable with herself! When she had finished with her eyebrows, not only had she reframed her eyes, she had also reframed her attitude. She was allowing softer and more vulnerable parts of herself to come out, parts that had most likely been locked up for a very long time.

DEFINING AND SOFTENING
YOUR LOOK
The purpose of making up your eyebrows is to add definition and to create a nice frame to the face. When I want to soften a woman's look, I start with the brows and then move to the lips. You don't naturally have peaks in either feature, so when you create them artificially, you're sending out a harsh, angry message. Why create a look that is contrary to your natural beauty?

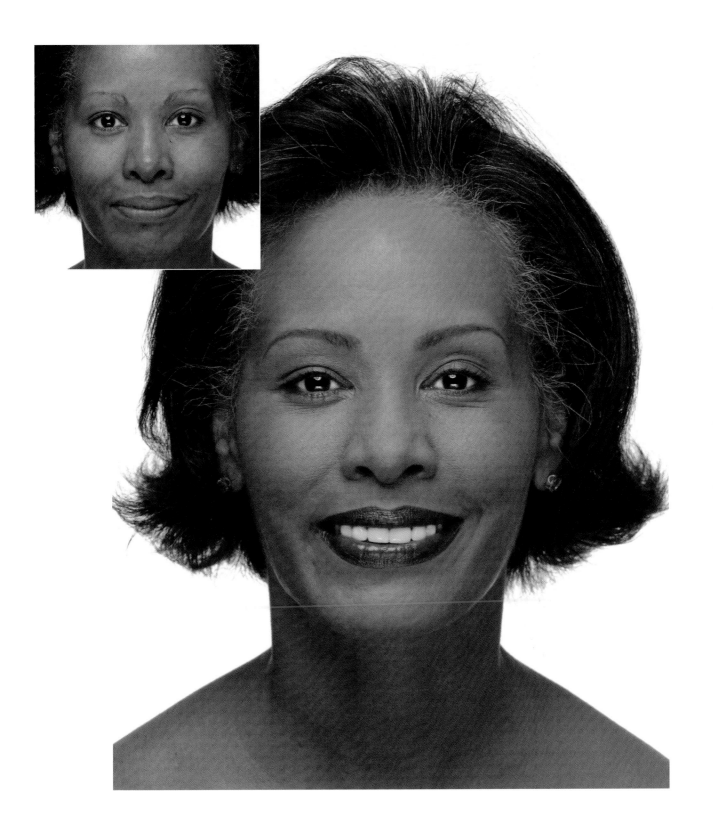

If your brows are sparse, too thin, too short, or shapeless, you can enhance them with an eyebrow pencil. A soft pencil, used in short, wispy strokes, will easily deposit color on the skin and brow hairs. Apply the strokes gently between the natural hairs in the direction in which your hair grows. Trying to simulate a hair with a hard, pointy pencil will result in a harsh, unnatural look.

After using your pencil, blend the strokes by brushing your brows in an upward direction. Smooth the top edge in the brow's natural direction. When you finish your entire makeup application, recheck your brows. If they need to be toned down, use your brush. If they need to be strengthened, add a little pencil. A light coat of clear mascara at this point will keep the brows in place. Clear mascara will also tame stray hairs that won't conform to the rest of the brow.

Let me add here that tinting and tattooing are other options. Tinting is done in many beauty salons so you can inquire. If you decide to have your brows tattooed, find a brow artist with a good reputation and make sure you see her work before you allow her to work on you. A bad tattoo job can ruin your look for a long time.

Things to remember about eyebrow color:

- The inner part of the brow should have the softest shade.

- If you intend to extend your eye makeup beyond the outer corner of your eye as in a more dramatic application, extend the eyebrow to keep the balance.

- You may not need color on your brows at all. Try a clear mascara on brows, then add color as needed.

GROOMING YOUR BROWS
Whether you choose to groom your brows to look dramatic or fuller, following the natural line of your own eyebrow is a good rule of thumb. In order to groom your brows and achieve the best framing results, you'll need three tools:

- A GOOD SET OF TWEEZERS. A professional pair of tweezers allows you to work fast with minimal pressure on the tool. This gives the instrument more longevity and makes it easier on you. I prefer the Tweezerman brand which is slightly more expensive than most of the competition, but the dependability is worth the investment. Some of the less expensive brands get old fast and when the points fail to make contact, you lose your ability to grasp the hair firmly. When your tweezers are in great condition, you can grasp the hair and pull quickly by the root without breaking it. If you break the hair follicle above the root, you'll get left with a tiny sprout of hair that you won't be able to get rid of until it grows out again.

- A BROW BRUSH OR A SOFT TOOTHBRUSH. I like using a two-sided brush with a comb on one side which can double as an eyelash separator. While natural bristles are much softer than nylon ones, they're also a little more expensive. If the extra expense is a burden, some women have found that using a soft child-size toothbrush is a good substitute. Just make sure the bristles aren't too wide to create a finely sculpted line. Once you've selected the right brush, it's important to keep it clean. To remove hair spray, oil, or brow makeup from the brush, I wash mine daily with a little eye makeup remover and a small amount of soap. Then I store it out in the open as you would a toothbrush, allowing the bristles to dry out in the air.

- A BROW PENCIL. One of my favorite tools in my makeup line is my taupe eyebrow pencil. I'm devoted to it because it works so well. The color is neutral, so whether I'm working on a blonde, brunette, or redhead, I can use the same taupe pencil, and adjust the shade with pressure rather than a different color. My taupe pencil accentuates the eyebrow itself, filling in sparseness between the hairs, leaving the brow looking like hair. The idea here is that you don't want to see the pencil line, you want to see the real hair of your brows. I also offer a brown pencil which I sometimes mix with the taupe for darker-skinned women, using a few strokes of each. I don't make a black brow pencil and I rarely use one, because it gives most women a very unnatural brow. We want to avoid the painted-on look. Always choose an eyebrow pencil with a very soft lead, so it doesn't drag against the skin. I find a long, slim pencil easier to control than a fat, stubby one.

TO TWEEZE OR NOT TO TWEEZE

Most of us need to tweeze, at least a little bit, to allow the brow to suggest a more finished look to the face. Besides the general rule of using a very good tweezer, it's a good idea to go to a reputable eyebrow professional at least once. It's worth the twelve to fifteen dollars to have her decide what's right for your face and establish the line for you. If economics or time limitations prevent you from returning, you can take over from there. In any event, take some time to figure out and establish the right shape for you, since your brows will frame the rest of your makeup and determine the message you're putting out.

A good way to "practice" the right shape is to draw it first. You can always wash off the pencil, try again, and then tweeze accordingly. When shaping brows, always think "up" and use your body type as a guide. If you're strong and athletic, a tiny brow will look out of sync with the rest of your body. Conversely, if you're small and delicate, a bushy brow will appear overpowering. Keep in mind that the shape you were born with is the best guide.

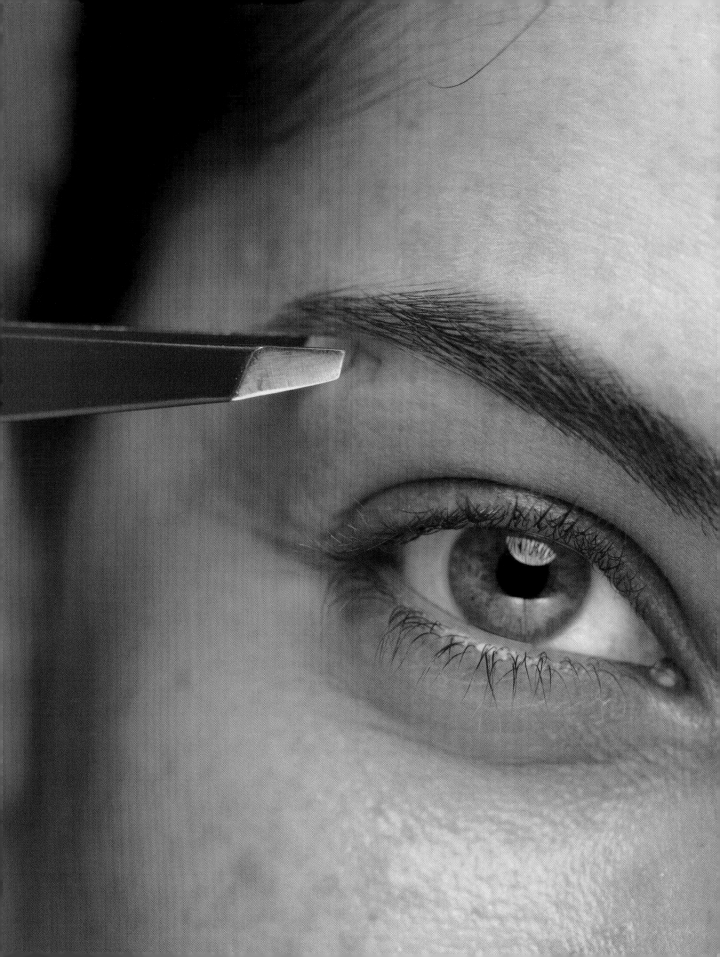

Since everyone's eyebrows are different, we all have to make adjustments as to where to begin and end the line of the brow. Always tweeze with good light so you can see well. If your eyebrow hairs are long, begin by trimming lightly with a manicure scissors. Start tweezing the hairs that grow across the nose area, between the brows. The brow should begin at an even angle with the inside of your eyes, and end just beyond the outer corner of your eye. Tweeze in a diagonal direction, starting on the inside, moving outward toward your ears. Allow the tail of the brow to extend past the outer corner of the eye.

To make it less painful, tweeze immediately after a warm shower. Applying a warm washcloth compress to the area will produce the same softening result. Always make sure the area is clean before you begin. Otherwise, you could get bumps and redness in the plucked area. For hypersensitive skin, try using a cream designed to numb teething babies' gums. If your skin gets red, apply ice immediately after tweezing.

By the way, don't tweeze too often. Once or twice a week should suffice. The idea is to control new growth so the brows don't lose their shape too quickly. Remember, shaving eyebrows can cause skin discoloration, and they never grow back the same. Save razors for other places not so delicate as the eye area. Tweezing requires adequate time, so don't pluck on the run. Follow these three steps for creating well groomed brows:

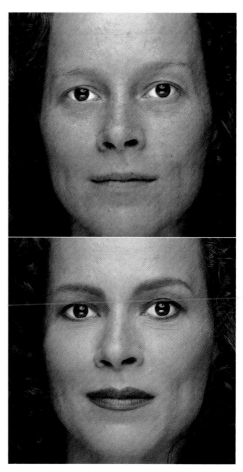

STEP #1: Your own eye will determine the line of your brow. To create a "V" shape, hold your brow pencil vertically along the side of the nose. One end should touch the outside of the nostril and the point should extend above the inner corner of the eye to the brow. This is the "beginning" of your brow. Any hairs that grow toward the middle beyond this point should be removed.

STEP #2: Keeping the end of the pencil fixed at the bottom of the nostril, shift the point toward the outside corner of the eye and extend it to the brow. This is the "end" of the brow. Remove any hairs growing beyond this point.

STEP #3: Looking straight ahead, extend the pencil vertically along the outside edge of the iris to the brow. This is the "middle" point where the arch should be.

If your brows need a trim, not a tweeze, use a small round-tipped scissors. Be careful; your brows grow back much more slowly than your bangs. To trim, follow these three steps:

STEP #1: Brush brows straight upward, and snip off any hairs that are overly long.

STEP #2: Brush brows straight downward and trim excess in the same way.

STEP #3: Brush brows into place. One by one, at random, snip any excess long hairs. Brush between each snip.

If you've lost your eyebrow hair for any reason, you'll need to draw in a brow. Use the brow bone as a guide. Find the area above your eye with your fingertips to establish where the forehead meets the eye socket. The brow usually grows along that ridge, so you can begin applying color there. Use a good, soft pencil, filling in the entire area with small strokes that end up resembling hair. Set the color in place with a light powder dusting.

As far as waxing goes, very few untrained people are adept at using hot wax, so it's better to stick to something you can control. I prefer tweezing, especially if you're doing it at home.

A few words on bleaching and dyeing:

Dyeing is nearly obsolete, because of the acidic content of dye around your eyes. If it needs to be done, go to a reputable professional.

Bleaching is far more popular, a process you can do yourself usually in conjunction with lightening your overall hair color. Buy the facial bleach used for upper lip hair, mix into a thick consistency, and leave it on for two minutes. If it burns or itches, remove bleach immediately and flush the area with water. Brunettes should know that too much bleach may look red.

Helpful hints:

- Don't overtweeze your brows. They won't look natural and they won't adequately accent your eyes. If you have to grow them out, be patient. It takes from three to six months for full regrowth.

- Work on brows alternately so you can keep them even.

- Draw the strokes between the natural hairs of your brow in the same direction they already grow.

- Never outline the brow and try to fill it in, even if you have no eyebrow hair. That looks really artificial!

- Brush your brows before and after applying makeup.

- A coat of dark mascara, brown or black, applied to the brows, will give you a dramatic evening look.

- Whether you're making up for daytime or evening, brows should never overpower your eyes.

- For women who have little or no eyebrow hair, tattooing may be an alternative. Make sure you seek out an expert in this field and be sure to view his or her past work.

BEAUTY MARK
1:

The eyebrows are the most important and expressive part of your face. Getting the right shape will help you to send the right message. If you can, it's important to do at least one initial consultation with an expert.

BEAUTY MARK
2:

The goal is a natural-looking brow, not something that looks drawn on.

BEAUTY MARK
3:

It may look as if your brow makeup is too heavy, but that can change with your eye makeup. Wait to make final brow adjustments until after you finish your eyes.

BEAUTY MARK
4:

When aging causes the eyelid to sag, the right brow shape will automatically open up the eyes.

APPLICATIONS for EYEBROWS

TO GROOM EYEBROWS

- Eyebrows create a natural frame for the eyes. Try not to change their natural shape.

- Beginning of eyebrow should be aligned with inner corner of eye and end just beyond.

- Arch is most important! It should be a soft arch (no peaks, a pointed or thin brow creates a harsh and/or surprised look on your face).

- Remember, brows are an expressive frame which sets the mood of your face.

1 Tweeze any hairs that obviously lie outside of your brow's natural shape. When removing a few hairs, alternate from one brow to the other. This eliminates over-tweezing and achieves a more balanced look.

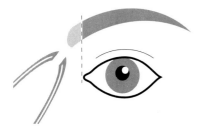

2 If a few hairs are missing, use taupe or brown pencil to draw in each hair. Begin at bottom of follicle and draw upward following hair direction. Use a light-handed fine stroke.

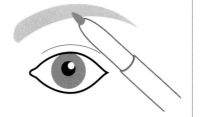

3 Brush eyebrow hairs up. Coat brush with damp soap on brow brush or spray brush with hair spray and brush through brows again to keep them up. For a groomed look, coat hairs instead with clear mascara. For a dramatic look, coat hairs with black mascara.

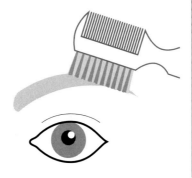

TO THICKEN THIN EYEBROWS

- Use brown or taupe eye pencil. Brown may be too harsh for women with lighter hair.

- Eyebrow should begin parallel to inner corner of eye and end just beyond eye.

- Eyebrow is fullest at nose bridge, gently arches, and softly tapers at end.

1 Start at nose bridge, use taupe or brown pencil and roll color over eyebrow hair.

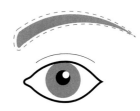

2 Deposit color again under eyebrow hairs, following natural shade. You can work under and slightly above natural hairs to thicken.

3 Blend with eyebrow brush, brush up hairs. Spray eyebrow brush with hair spray or apply damp soap, and brush through hairs to keep brows brushed up. Try coating eyebrows with clear mascara for a fresh look.

TO THICKEN SPARSE EYEBROWS

- To strengthen the natural frame for eyes use taupe or brown eye pencil (for lighter-haired women, brown may be too harsh).

- Use natural brow shape as a guide.

- Beginning of eyebrow should be parallel with inner corner of eye and end just beyond eye.

1 Using the taupe or brown eyebrow pencil, draw in individual hairs between your natural hairs. Start each stroke from base upward, following natural hair direction. Use a light-handed, fine stroke.

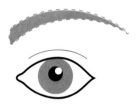

2 Roll pencil under eyebrow to deposit color on skin to thicken brow shape. Make sure you follow natural eyebrow shape. Brow should be fullest at nose bridge, gently arching and softly tapering at the ends. Using eyebrow brush, brush through brow with upward sweep. You can deposit damp soap on brush or spray it with hair spray, then brush through eyebrow again, keep sweeping up.

3 For a groomed look, instead of soap or hair spray, coat eyebrow hairs and brush up with my clear gel mascara. If drama is your look, try coating eyebrow hairs lightly with my black mascara.

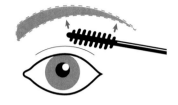

FULL EYEBROWS

- The beginning of the eyebrow should be in line with inner corner of the eye and end just beyond eye.

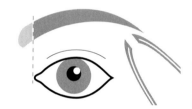

1 Tweeze hairs on nose bridge (if any). Remove only hairs which are obviously outside of the natural shape. When tweezing, remove a few hairs from one eye, then alternate to other brow. This eliminates overtweezing and achieves a more balanced look. Using the eyebrow brush, brush hairs up. If a few hairs are missing, draw in each hair using a light feather-touch stroke. Begin at bottom and draw upward following hair direction.

2 To keep brow hairs swept up deposit damp soap on eyebrow brush, or spray hair spray on eyebrow brush, and brush through eyebrows.

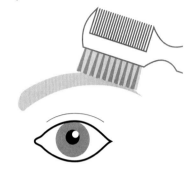

3 For a fresh look, coat eyebrows with clear mascara. For a more dramatic look, try coating brows lightly with black mascara.

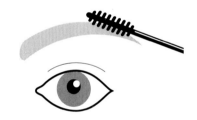

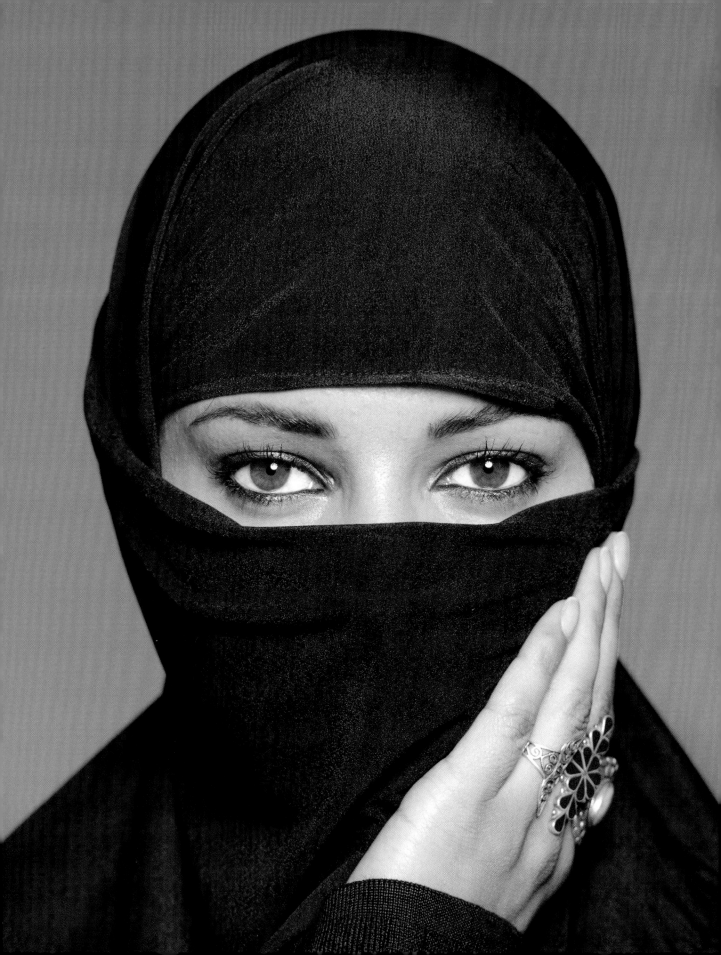

7: EYES WIDE OPEN

THE ULTIMATE COMMUNICATORS You can learn a lot by looking into someone's eyes. People call them windows to the soul because everything is said through the eyes. The eyes are the communication centers of the face.

I don't believe in trying to change the look of your eyes with makeup dramatically. It won't work, and your eyes should be communicators, not an advertising campaign for the brand of makeup you've chosen. Makeup applied well will intensify beautiful eyes, even if you look great without makeup. Of course, I'm referring to a natural application that will enhance the true color of your eyes and make them look more open.

In the sixties and seventies, women tried copying exaggerated eye styles with liner. They thought they were communicating a sense of high fashion, but really, I think it was all about imitating someone else. Today, liner is all about defining the eyes as they are, not making them look like they belong to somebody else's face. Playing up the unique look of your particular eyes is the goal.

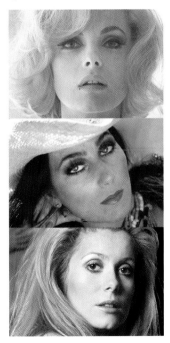

I consider eyes to be the quintessential beauty signature of every woman's face, no matter what color or shape yours might be. Don't get stuck thinking your eyes have to be huge, almond-shaped, or perfectly spaced in order to be considered "pretty." There are no perfect eyes, they all have their individual beauty. I've never seen a pair that weren't remarkably lovely.

This is where makeup can serve you by enhancing the beauty that's already there. When you feel secure that your eyes look fantastic and are well made up, you'll be more likely to look directly at someone. That adds up to better communication with your friends and your business associates.

DIFFERENT STROKES FOR DIFFERENT FOLKS

Shadows, liner, and mascara work together to enhance the eyes. An application of subtle color will make your natural eye color appear more intense and create the illusion of longer, lusher eyelashes. Makeup can also make the eyes look larger, which most women find desirable.

Different eye types:

If your eyes are **small** in proportion to your face, that doesn't mean they aren't just as attractive as larger ones. Most likely, you also have delicate features, and so makeup can make your eyes look larger and more dramatic. Remember, though, that too much shadow and liner will make them look smaller. Good placement and blending are important here.

If your eyes are **large** and tend to dominate your face, correct placement of makeup will help them look not overly made-up. Balance is the key. If your makeup is strong, your lips need to be strong also. If your makeup is pale or your eyes are bare, a muted lipstick will balance out that look.

Downturned eyes are extremely versatile. You can go without makeup for a more innocent look, or you can use shadow and liner to counteract the downturn. Apply your shadow at the outside corner, blending in toward the center, to give the eye a subtle lift.

I've seen women with eyes set so **deep**, no lid shows when the eyes are open, but this doesn't stop the eyes from being the central focus of the face. If this describes you, a bit of foundation on the lid that's one-half to one shade lighter than you use on the rest of your face will help to define the lid. Wearing shadow above the crease of the lid instead of hiding it on the lid itself, is a good way to experiment.

If you have very little space between the inner corners of your eyes and the bridge of your nose, you have what we call **close-set** eyes. If you wish your eyes to look a little wider, emphasizing the outer corners with shadow will create a wonderfully dramatic effect.

Wide-set eyes means there is a larger than usual space between the inside corners and the bridge of the nose. Making up the inner corners of the eye will treat the wideness as an asset.

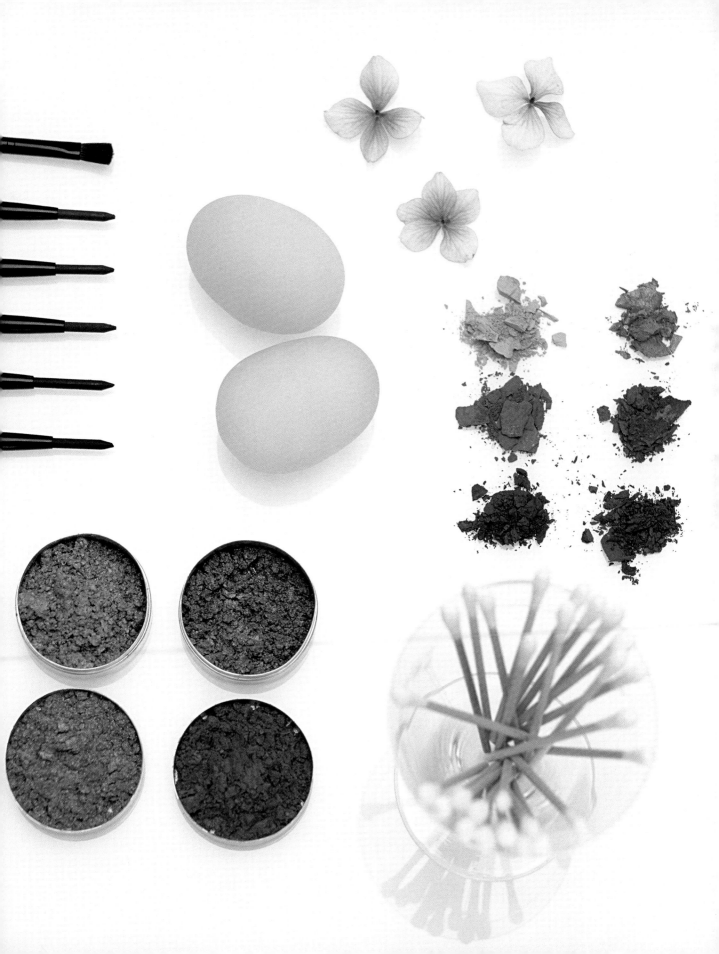

LINING YOUR EYES

Since liner is all about defining the eyes as they are, not making them look like they belong on somebody else's face, playing up the unique look of your particular eyes is the goal.

Keep the liner color natural. I'm not saying that you can't use greens and purples if you want to. I have brown and black in my basic kit, but I also have fine wine colors in my burgundy color kit, and an eye pencil that will coordinate with burgundy, brown, or black. These fun colors are best used when you're accenting or adding interest to a specific look. The goal is to exaggerate the natural definition of your eyes, so start with basic browns before you add color. I also recommend smudging a dark brown, (or in some cases, black) liner, to soften the look.

There are several kinds of liner available in the marketplace: felt-tip, liquid, and pencil. When using felt-tip, shake it to urge out the color, and try it on your hand first to check the thickness. Do that second step with liquid, too. A good brush is essential for liquid application, so make sure the brush does the trick. If the enclosed one doesn't, purchase a good brush separately. For an even liquid application, dip the tip of the brush in the liner, wetting it slightly, then testing it. With liquid, do not smudge.

I prefer a pencil liner to a liquid or felt-tip. I find that pencil creates a more natural look, I can blend with the soft lead more easily, and I can apply it lower into the lash line. When you use pencil liner, always make sure it isn't rough on your skin. This area is so delicate, you need to take special care not to cause irritation.

A good trick to line the eyes is to look downward into a mirror. This allows you to see the whole eyelid while you make it up. Practicing when you don't have an important event will help give you confidence.

To line the eye, start on the lower lid, just beneath the lashes. At the outside corner, draw a line that extends about two-thirds of the way toward the inner corner. If your skin is loose in this area, gently hold the outer corner of the eye slightly taut to make the skin smooth. When you're finished, always smudge the line with your sponge. Stay as close to the lash line as possible. On the upper lid, draw a line from the inner corner to the outer corner, thickening the line toward the outer corner. Again, get as close as possible to the lash line.

> *I am a sergeant in the US Navy, assigned as a medic. I was a little skeptical about your choice of pinks and browns in the eyeshadow kit, but the colors made my green eyes really come out. I also want you to know that your makeup techniques are so efficient, I can come home from Physical Training, take a shower, put on your makeup, do my hair, get dressed in my camouflage fatigues, and eat breakfast, all in 60 minutes.*
>
> —*Sgt. P.C., Ft. Polk, LA*

Avoid using too much liner. This will create rings of blackness around your eyes, a throw back to the late sixties and early seventies. This look is dated and will make your face appear hard and tired. A lightly smudged line will allow the true color of the iris to predominate, creating a contemporary and natural look.

Whichever form of liner you decide to use, remember that eyeliner not only defines the eyes, it also helps give the illusion of thicker eyelashes.

IN SHADING, LESS IS MORE
The purpose of eye shadow is to highlight and define your eyes. It also expresses your moods and your creativity. Shadow can create perception, so adding a darker color in the crease right below the brow bone will give the illusion of more depth by recessing your eye. A darker color over the lidded area of the eye will make it appear smaller, while a lighter color in the center of the eyelid will open it. That's what shadow is all about—creating depth in order to bring out the beauty of your eyes. I encourage experimentation, so forget "seasonal" color palettes. As long as you're enhancing your beauty, I believe that less is more. Accessible eyes, open and deep, is a beautiful look we can create with the right application of makeup.

When I'm choosing a shadow color, I look first at a woman's eyes, and then I go deeper, noticing the flecks of color in her irises. Whatever I see deep inside the eye is what I want to build on. Think about making the eye color "pop." For example, brown eyes might be flecked with gold or green. A blue eye might also be flecked with smoky gray as well as gold, green, lavender, or turquoise. Matching blues to a blue eye will fade out your eye color. Green and hazel irises often have flecks of pale gray, turquoise, gold, or dark brown. Matching greens will fade eye color.

If a woman has a particular shade of blonde hair, I might avoid a gold shadow that would wash out her hair color. I'd play up the smoky gray, instead. The idea here, instead of being obvious, is to bring out colors in your eyes that somebody else might be missing. Then you're accenting who you are and playing up what you have, rather than competing with Mother Nature.

This doesn't mean you can't have fun playing with color. I have shimmer in my line for evenings (which women love), and rich, wonderful shadow colors to create all kinds of different looks. For instance, if you're wearing an outfit with three shades of color running through it, you can accent one of them with an eye shade. Choosing all three would be somewhat confusing, though. It's about complementing and creating interest. If I choose a blue eye shadow, I take the edge off by mixing it with a softer color, which is why I put several complementary shades in my shadow compacts.

The things to keep in mind when choosing shadows are as follows:

- FINISH: This describes a matte or a more shiny look. Matte is considered more classic, while shimmer is nice for special occasions like fancy evenings or black tie events.

- TEXTURE: Choose a shadow that is silky smooth and blends easily over your skin. Avoid grainy and scratchy shadows that look dry and cakey.

- INTENSITY: The more pigment in a shadow, the darker the color, and vice versa. If you put on several layers of shadow and still can't bring the color up to the intensity you want, there simply isn't adequate pigment in the product to achieve your goal.

Remember: If you wear contact lenses or you have extremely sensitive eyes, shimmer (created by mica) may cause flakes to fly into your eyes, which results in redness and irritation.

Applying eye shadow takes three quick steps:

- STEP #1: After you establish the outer corner of your eye, apply a medium or light shade in a ">" shape and blend it toward the center of your lid.

- STEP #2: Add a lighter shade to the inner corner of your eye and blend with the previous shade.

- STEP #3: Apply a darker shade at your lash line on the outside corner and blend into ">" and into crease.

For downturned eyes, adjust the "<" so its point angles upward. Blend the darker shade on the outer third of the lid only. Blend the lighter shade in the inner corner of the lid, up into brow. Make sure both shades are blended well, starting at crease and moving up to the brow bone. No lines of demarcation.

Remember: You can use only one color if you choose. Use a maximum of two shades that blend together and compliment each other. This means no harsh edges or lines of demarcation. For all the following examples, one to two shades of color for highlighting and shadowing will work fine.

SHADOW TIPS:

- Light shadow on the lids, as opposed to dark ones, will look best as they cause the eyes to open rather than recede. Always use colors that blend with each other in a natural way.

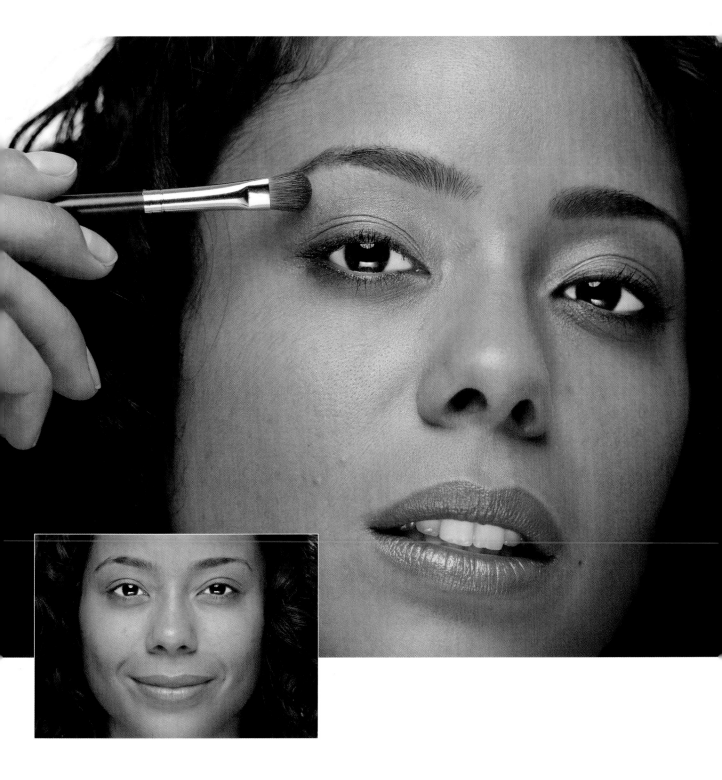

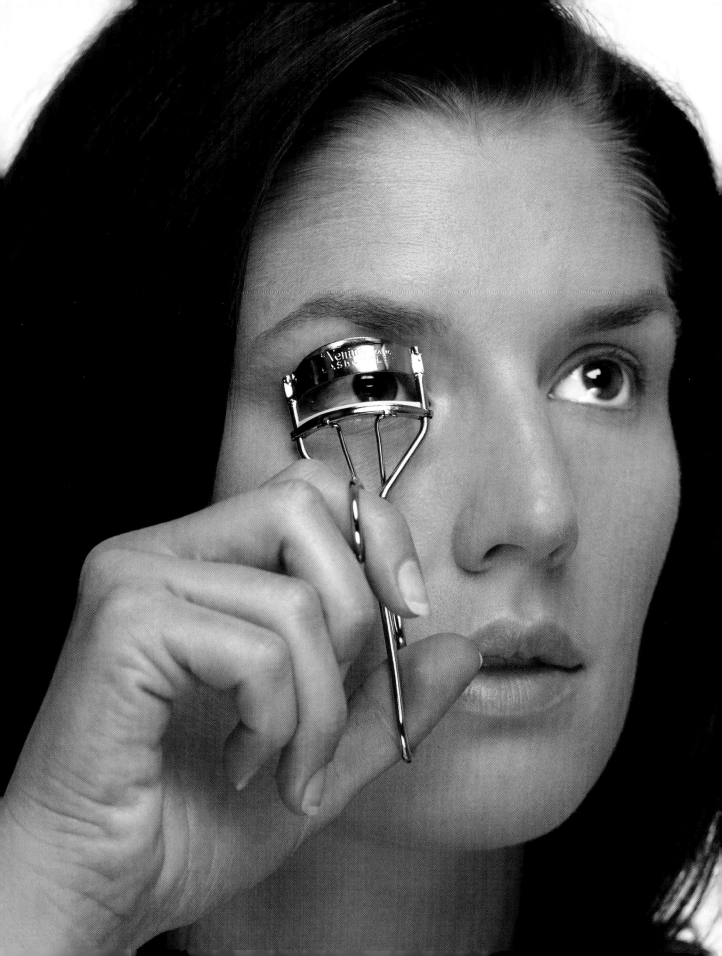

- Your natural skin tone has an impact on how the shadow looks. Be careful with dark shades, especially if you have light skin. Very dark skin may require rich, saturated shades.

- Always keep shimmer subtle. Shiny textures, although they're fun, will highlight imperfections and wrinkles, so be cautious.

- The skin area around the eye is usually the first to show age. If upper lids are "hooded," a light touch of shadow can help.

THE POWER OF MASCARA Putting on mascara is the point in a makeup application when it all comes together. This is true with makeovers for my infomercials and with my celebrity clients, who I'm proud to say include such great beauties as brilliant news anchor, Barbara Walters, and countless talented actors, among them Kate Jackson, Kathleen Turner, and Rosanna Arquette; as well as musicians Carly Simon and Reba McIntyre, and so many more. Though I've worked with such diverse legends as Bette Davis, Ringo Starr, and Jimmy Stewart, nowhere was the power of mascara more apparent than when I did my makeup classes at Sybil Brand Correctional Institute.

When the class was over and I got ready to leave, mascara was the only item the inmates were allowed to keep. These women, stripped of literally everything else, treasured this one small gift so much, I started thinking about mascara as a magic wand we could wave and change the way we think and feel about ourselves. It's truly magic when you see a woman open this little tube, apply it to her eyelashes, and suddenly gain a kind of power over herself. It's as if she pumped the wand and became stronger. I know women who are comfortable going out with almost no makeup, except a little mascara. It's no wonder that mascara is the number one selling item in the entire cosmetic industry.

I've seen mascara make a woman's face really come alive, time and time again, when I was working as a makeup artist. It's like a wake-up call, the turning point in the process of a makeover, when a woman comes out of her shell and starts to feel better about herself. Whether she wants me to put the mascara on for her or she prefers to do it herself, this is usually the point where she starts to feel in control and more comfortable with herself.

When curling your eyelashes, do so before you apply your mascara. Just make sure you go slowly, so you don't catch that delicate eyelid skin in the curler. If you wait to curl until after mascara, you'll weaken your eyelashes and break them off. Ten to twenty seconds is sufficient with a good eyelash curler.

75

Mascara originally was packaged as a cream in a teeny little tube. You'd open a container that looked like a matchbox, and inside you'd find a tube of makeup and a tiny brush. Later, it was packaged as a powder. You'd have to wet the brush and apply it. Today, along with these other methods, we've found the easiest way to present it and to apply it, as a magic wand you pump into the tube and roll it on.

Thick, dark lashes are considered sensual, so we all seem to go for mascara, even if we wear no other makeup. The purpose of mascara is three-fold: lengthening, thickening, and conditioning. Most mascaras are made up of pigments, waxes, and oils, so when choosing your brand, think about what you want to accomplish. Since we don't all have eyelashes like my son, Jackson, we can use all the help we can get.

Here are some guidelines:

- Cake mascara is a dry, thick powder to which you add water and apply with a brush. It gives a good, thick look to the lashes, but it's quite tricky to apply and it takes a special solvent to remove it.

- Water soluble mascara, my makeup of choice, can be removed with water. Although it will run in the wake of tears, rain, or a swimming pool, it generally has good staying power and has the widest range of choices and effects. I suggest you use this under normal circumstances.

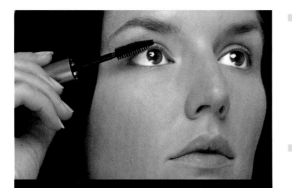

Most people don't know that 68 percent of cosmetic users buy mascara. But mascara may well be the equivalent of the VCR: Nearly everyone has it: next to no one really knows how to use it to its full potential.

—Allure *magazine, August, 1999*

- Waterproof mascara doesn't come off in rain or with tears. It gives a thick look to the lashes, but removing it is difficult. It contains ingredients that can dry and break the lashes, so I suggest you use it only when necessary. Like cake, it also needs a special solvent to be removed.

- Clear mascara contains little or no pigment. It creates a glossy look which can be placed underneath a color to create a thicker look. Used alone, it will enhance the gloss of your lashes, so it's great for teens.

After curling the lashes, coat them with a layer of mascara. Start by rolling the wand from root to tip, moving the lashes in an upward motion. Let it dry and then comb your lashes to avoid residue. Now apply one more layer, let it dry and comb. Do the bottom lashes with less mascara on the wand to avoid clumping. The whole process is simple, it takes a few seconds, and it makes all the difference in the world. If you want to create a different, more open look to your face, you can try not making up the bottom lashes.

By the way, if your eyelashes are short, apply mascara at the roots, using a long stroke first, and then lift the wand to move the lashes upward at the tip. You can even train the lashes upward with your fingers if need be, but be careful not to stab yourself in the eye. A fuller brush will deposit color which will add more density to your lashes, giving a thicker, more luxurious illusion.

HELPFUL HINTS:

- Define the eye with a natural brown eyeliner before you add color accents.

- The purpose of shadow is to highlight and redefine your eyes.

- It's always more awkward to do the opposite eye. Right-handed women should do the left, more difficult eye first, while your hand is less tired.

- Begin applying shadow at the outer corner of the eye and work inward. This method deposits the most color near the outer corner and makes the eye appear larger.

- Begin lining lash line from outer corner to where lashes end, moving toward the nose.

- If you wear contact lenses, put them in before applying mascara or any other makeup around your eyes.

- Curl eyelashes *before* applying mascara to avoid lashes breaking off.

- When shopping for mascara, you need not only a great brush, but a great formula, that's neither too wet nor too dry. Look for the perfect formula for you.

- If it seems like your mascara is smudging, you may be using a formula that's too wet.

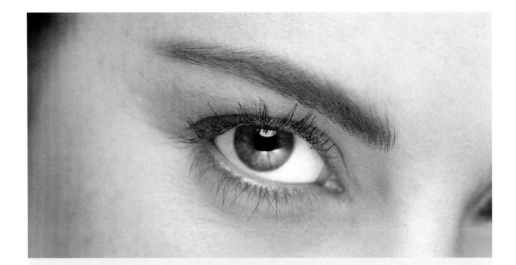

BEAUTY MARK

1:

When choosing shadow color, look deep inside the eye at the flecks on the iris.

BEAUTY MARK

2:

Smudge eyeliner with sponge for a shadowy effect.

BEAUTY MARK

3:

For final adjustments to eye makeup, look straight into the mirror with your eyes open naturally.

BEAUTY MARK

4:

Make sure to remove all your makeup completely each night before sleep. You'll wake up with healthier skin that will look clean and fresh when you go to apply your makeup for the day.

APPLICATIONS for EYES

TO ENLARGE SMALL EYES

1 Start at outer corner of eye with medium tone shadow. Set shape by angling slightly upward. Apply shadow color on entire eyelid as far as crease, blending outward.

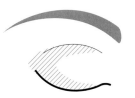

2 Softly blend darkest color in crease and at outer corner of eye.

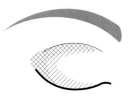

3 Line upper lid at lash line from inner corner to outer corner.

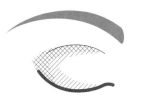

4 Line lower lid under lashes on outer corner only, about one third of eye from outer corner.

5 Apply mascara.

TO WIDEN CLOSE-SET EYES

1 Using lightest shade of eye shadow, apply to one-half of eyelid, from inner corner to center.

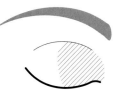

2 Blend darker tone on outer corner of eye, blending outward to elongate and to soften.

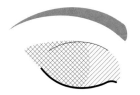

3 Blend darker tone from middle of lid upward to brow bone, extend beyond outer eye corner, drawing eyes further apart.

4 Add highlight under brow. Add lighter color on outer eye to soften dark shadow.

5 Line top of eye at lash line on outer two-thirds, which pulls the eye outward. Do not add liner on inner third near corner of eyes, which will bring eyes closer together.

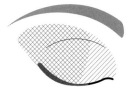

6 Line lower lid under lashes starting in the middle and working to outside corner.

7 Smudge pencil line down to just a shadow for a smoky look, which is great for evening.

8 Apply mascara.

HOODED EYES

1. With a medium to dark shadow color, start at outer corner of eyes and set shape slightly upward.

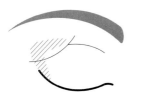

2. Blend darker shade over hooded area, extending it into brow bone.

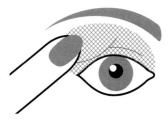

3. Blend medium tone in center of lid, softly blending to soften brow bone.

4. Use lightest shade in corner of eyelid. Highlight just under brow with lightest shade. Do not extend highlight too far down, keeping it at brow to emphasize hood.

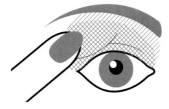

5. Line upper eyelid from inner corner of eye to outer corner. Keep line as close as possible to lash line.

6. Starting at outer corner, line lower lid under lashes, only lining one-third of bottom of the eye.

7. Smudge pencil line until just a shadow.

8. Apply mascara.

WIDE-SET EYES

1. Start at outer corner of eye with medium tone shadow. Set shape by angling slightly upward. Apply shadow color on entire eyelid as far as crease, blending outward.

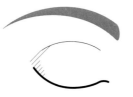

2. Blend medium-light toned shadow to brow bone, and blend to center of lid. Do not extend shadow outward.

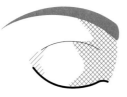

3. Blend darker color in corner of eye on lid, working softly along side of bridge of nose into fullest area of brow.

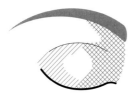

4. Blend darker color from inner corner to center of eyelid, blending into medium shade that started from outer corner.

5. Concentrate lightest shade in center under brow. Do not add lightest shade to outer edges under brow, which would pull eye outward.

6. Line upper eyelid at lash line moving from very inner corner to outward corner.

7. Line under lower lid with taupe and brown or black. Line outer one-half with taupe, then line one-half or one-fourth beyond taupe with brown or black to pull eye into nose.

8. Smudge pencil line down to just a shadow for a smoky effect.

9. Apply mascara.

ROUND EYES

1. Using a medium to dark shade in outer corner, shape slightly upward.

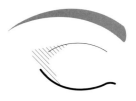

2. Continue medium to dark shade, blending inward along brow bone. Shade three-fourths of brow, then STOP! Do not shade last fourth with this color.

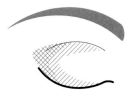

3 Blend lighter shade in corner of eye on lid.

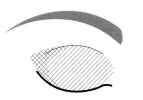

4 Use medium shade on lid in very center.

5 Line upper eyelid at lash line from inner corner to outer corner.

6 Thicken outer corner liner and slightly fade slant upward. You can blend this down with your foundation sponge. This extends eyes outward, counteracting the roundness.

7 Line under lower lashes on the outer one-third from outside corner of eye.

8 Smudge pencil line down to just a shadow for smoky effect.

9 Apply mascara.

PROMINENT EYES

1 Start medium shade of shadow in outer eye. Do not overextend.

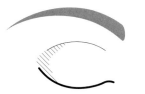

2 Use medium to dark shade of shadow all over upper eyelid to brow-bone.

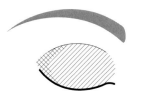

3 Blend lighter shade below brow, blending into brow-bone color.

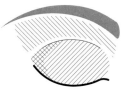

4 Line entire upper lid at lash line, smudge line softly with cotton swab so there are no hard lines, just a soft muted shadow.

5 Line under lower lashes one-half way, starting from outer eye corner working to center.

6 Smudge pencil line to shadow for smoky effect.

7 Apply mascara.

DEEP-SET EYES

1 Use medium shade of shadow starting at corner of eye, slightly angling upward, and blend.

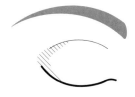

2 Use medium light shade on entire eyelid. Blend softly to brow bone.

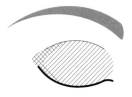

3 Blend lightest shade in center of eyelid to open up eye.

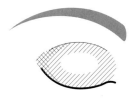

4 Blend lightest shade under brow.

5 Stay away from dark colors on brow bone, which will make deep set eyes look even deeper. Stay away from eyeliner on top lids, which will sink eyes further back.

6 Line lower lid under lashes on outer one-third.

7 Smudge pencil line to just a shadow to counter heaviness of top brow.

8 Apply mascara.

DROOPY EYES

Keep eyes open during application for better placement to drooping area.

1. Using a medium shade of shadow, start at outer corner and shape the eye upward to counter droopiness. Blend on outer one-third of lid, never blending downward.

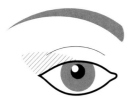

2. Blend lighter shade into corner of lid, softly blending up, following along the sides of the nose into brow.

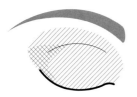

3. Apply a darker shade in center crease at brow bone, blending into lighter color toward nose and slightly blending to medium color at outer corner.

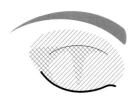

4. Keep darkest shade in center of eye, as darker shade in outer corner will emphasize droopiness.

5. Line upper eye at lash line starting from inner corner outward. Do not line end of outer corner, which will pull eyes downward. Keep one-eighth from outer corner unlined.

6. Line lower lid under lashes starting from outer corner and continuing three-fourths of full eye.

7. Smudge pencil line down to just a shadow, making sure outer corner of lower lid is very smudged. Keep darkest concentration in center.

8. Apply mascara

EYELINING

- Thin line at lashes thickens appearance of lashes.

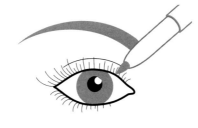

- Hold outside corner of eye with fingertip when applying.
- Thick line at lashes gives more drama.
- Always blend line with wedge-sponge or cotton swab to soften.
- Make sure pencil is sharpened.
- If you have dark shadows under your eyes, stay away from bottom lining, which emphasizes shadows.

1. Begin lining lash from outer corner to where lashes end toward nose.

2. Connect inner corner of eye to lash line by drawing on inside edge of skin.

3. Smudge lines with wedge sponge or cotton swab.

4. For a minimal lower line effect, dot between lashes with pencil.

APPLYING MASCARA

- Before applying mascara, if your lashes are straight, curl upper lashes with an eyelash curler. Make sure you fit all lash hairs in curler and curler is fitted as close as possible to the base of lash.

- For a no makeup look, coat under and lower lashes with clear mascara only, remember to comb lashes with eyebrow brush/comb application.

1. Coat lashes with brown or black mascara from very base to lash tips with full strokes.

2. Also apply by sweeping from top side down as well as coating under the lashes. Close eyes, apply from roots to tips.

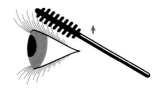

3 Comb through lashes with comb side of eyebrow brush to separate. It's easiest before they have dried. Repeat after each application of mascara.

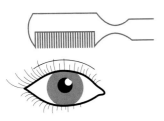

4 Hold brush parallel to nose, coat bottom lashes with tip of mascara brush.

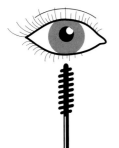

5 Comb through bottom lashes with eyebrow comb/brush.

6 To lengthen top lashes further, after lashes have dried, coat lash tips two or three times with black mascara (drying and separating between applications).

7 Lash base must be coated as close to the flesh as possible, which defines the eye shape and keeps application looking natural.

8 For the thickest lashes, coat upper and lower lashes with clear mascara; comb through, then coat upper and lower lashes as described above with black mascara.

APPLICATION TIPS YOU NEED TO KNOW

- Although adult women enjoy the look of shimmery, iridescent eye shadow, it emphasizes lines, wrinkles, and sagging lids. Instead, define the eyes with a matte shade, to create a smoother, glamorous look.

- Paying attention to your eyebrows, which frame your eyes, will make a significant difference in your appearance.

- Adding color in the eye rim closes down the eye, making it appear smaller. Place liner underneath the bottom lashes to create the illusion of larger, smokier eyes.

- Color beneath the lower eyelashes tends to fight with eye color, and to emphasize puffy eyes and dark circles.

- Avoid starting application of eye shadow at inner corner of eye and working back toward the outside, as that will sweep the eye downward. Instead, work eye shadow from outside corner and move it inward, setting eye shade without casting outside eye corner downward.

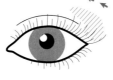

- If you have blue or green eyes, stay away from shadow colors that match too closely to your own eye color. It will detract from the color of your eyes. Look deep inside the iris and match the flecks instead.

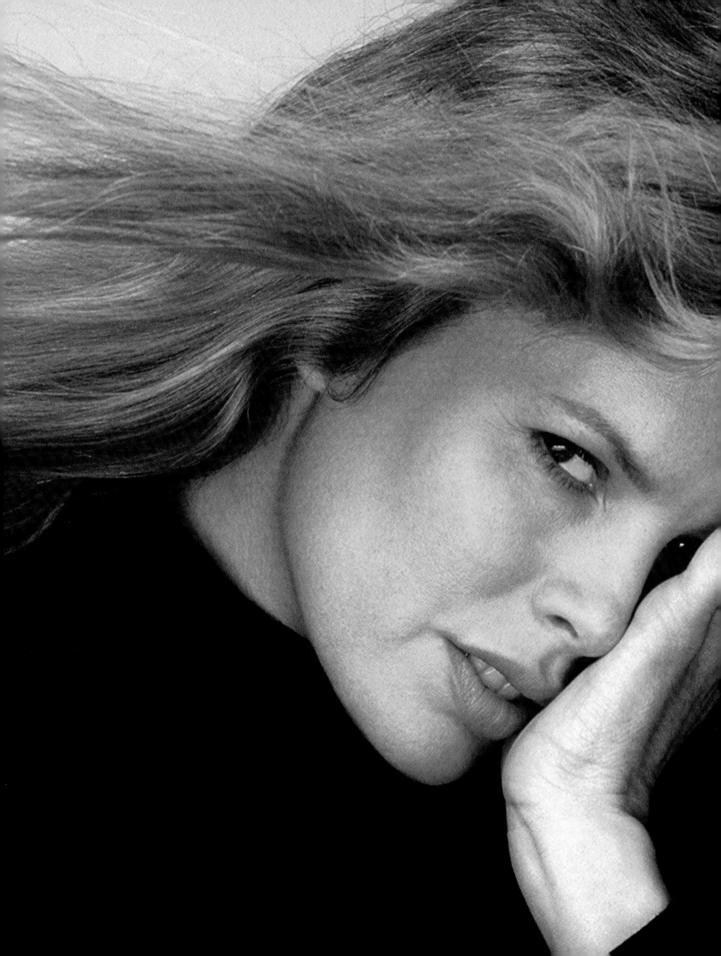

BLUSH: A NATURAL GLOW

THE "FEEL GOOD" BEAUTY SECRET

Brides and babies have a natural glow to their cheeks. The rest of us could use some blush. I depend on it to make a difference in my appearance, especially when the stress begins to show on my face. Toward evening, when I feel washed out and need a lift, but I don't have time to do a complete touch-up, I like to add some color to my cheeks. It's a pick-me-up. It makes me feel better and puts some life back into my face, even when I don't feel that sparkle. That's why I call blush the "feel good" secret, an exciting part of the makeup process. Applied correctly, blush can make you look healthier and more vibrant, qualities that are contagious, because when you look better, you feel better, too.

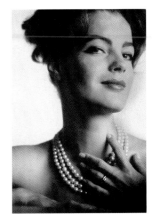

Today, most women use blush to create a natural glow. Think about it. When you're happy or working out, you get a natural flush of color in your cheeks. Follow your own lead and use blush to accentuate what's beautiful about you, not to change the way you look. Remember, blush is not for doing liposuction on your face because you think the shape is wrong or you were given the wrong kind of cheekbones. Part of accepting who you are is accepting the natural shape of your face. Who said sunken cheekbones were better than full ones?

FINDING THE APPLE

So many women ask me where the blush goes, and I know it can be confusing. At first, I wasn't so sure myself. After all, since all women have different shaped faces, doesn't the blush go in different places? I finally realized that the shape of a person's face has nothing to do with placement of blush. Here's a good way to figure it out:

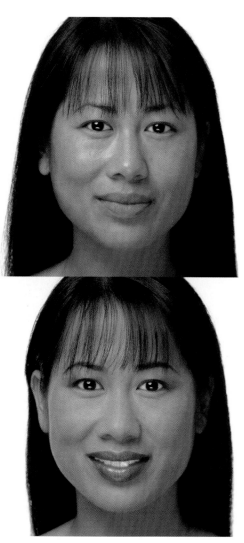

I like to use two blush shades, lighter and darker, that blend well for each makeup application, one for definition and light contouring, and another for highlighting. Remember, *no heavy contouring with dark colors*. One of the hardest things to do with blush is to take weight off your face, so don't try. You may end up doing the opposite. It's all about adding a healthy, natural glow.

With your fingers, locate the joint where the upper jaw meets the lower. This is the beginning of your cheekbone. Trace the bone with your finger until you can feel a natural hollow. (Yes, it's there for everyone, whether your cheekbones are high or low.) Apply the slightly darker tone of blush just beneath this bone, beginning in the hollow. Start with a subtle layer of the darker tone of blush beneath the cheekbones, maybe a half-tone darker than the rest of your face. With one smooth stroke, make a "C" shape up toward your temple and hairline.

The lighter shade goes on the "apple" of your cheek. Just smile at yourself in the mirror, something you should be getting good at by now. The fleshy part of your cheekbone, the area that pillows up, is the apple. Swirl your brush into the blush powder. Shake off excess powder. Gently apply blush in a sweeping motion on the apple from the center of your face in an upward direction. For a more natural look, don't make it apparent where the blush begins and ends and don't stray too low with the brush. That will make your face look heavy at your jawbone. Think up, not down. And remember—always apply and blend. Then blend again.

Remember to finish your eyes before you apply blush. When your eyes are done, you won't feel the need for as much

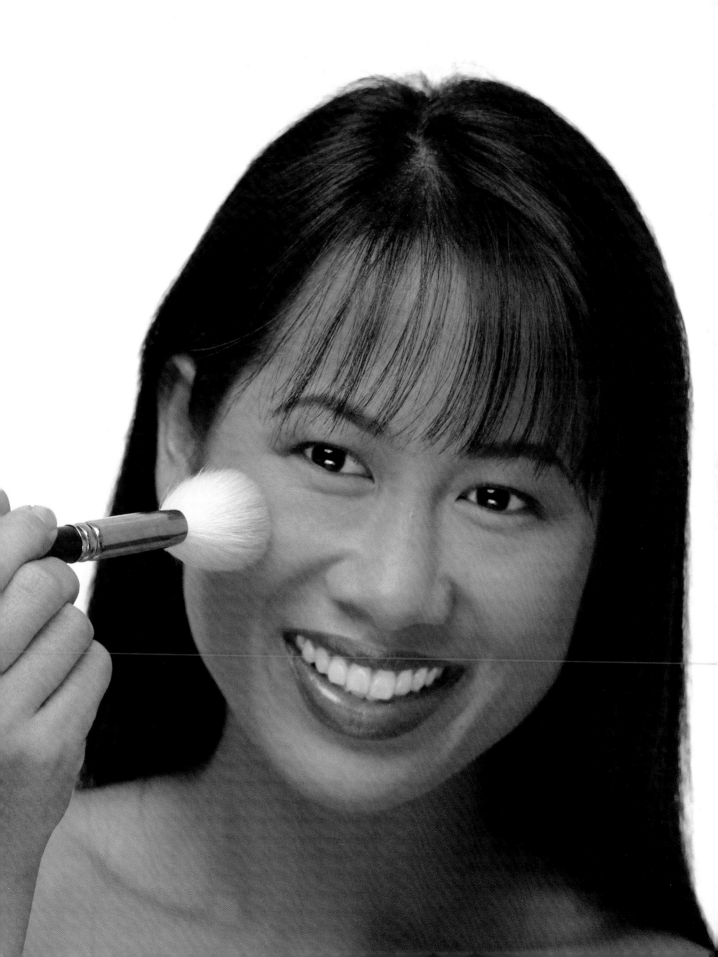

color on your cheeks and you probably won't overdo it. Start with a small amount of blush, finish your makeup, and then go back and add more if necessary. It's important to keep in mind that you always want to use an ultra-light touch. Once again, no tugging or pulling at your skin. That can be damaging, especially with older skin that has lost some of that youthful elasticity.

GENERAL BLUSH APPLICATION GUIDELINES:

- In a complete makeup application, blush comes after the eyes. With your eyes nicely defined, you won't have the tendency to overdo blush.

- Use two shades that blend well together. The lighter shade goes on the apple of the cheek, the darker goes beneath the cheekbone. Think subtle, especially with the darker tone.

- Start with a very light touch. You can always add more later, if necessary.

- For too heavy an application, use that trusty old sponge, gently blending away excess.

- Blend thoroughly. Stripes and circles are "out"!

- Make sure you've blended the blush so it fades completely into the hairline.

WHICH SHAPE ARE YOU?

LONG FACE You have the choice either to emphasize the length or to add width. The first option is dramatic, in which you would use a smaller amount of makeup, maybe a touch of eyeliner, some mascara, and a bold, shiny lipstick, with no blush at all. This will look best with hair slicked back away from the face. For a softer look, place a light shade of blush on the top of the cheekbone and a darker shade beneath. Most of the color goes on the outer edges of the bone right where the jaws meet, and then upward toward the temple. To shorten the look of the face, bangs or soft waves on the forehead work wonders.

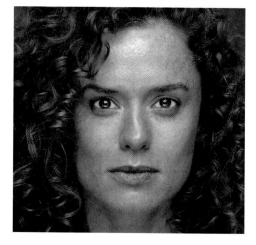

When applying, use the darker color in a "C," concentrating color at outer edge of the face, which should be the middle of the "C" and up toward the temple. Add your lighter shade above the cheekbone and blend. Dust the lighter shade on the apple.

LONG FACE TIPS:

- Highlight the cheekbones and widen the face with two blush shades.

- Apply blush low on temple, never moving higher up than the tip of the eyebrows.

- Be careful not to place blush too close to the under-eye area, or it will look puffy.

- No blush on forehead or chin. Keep attention focused on eyes and lips.

- To highlight the center of the face, lightly dust the tip of the nose.

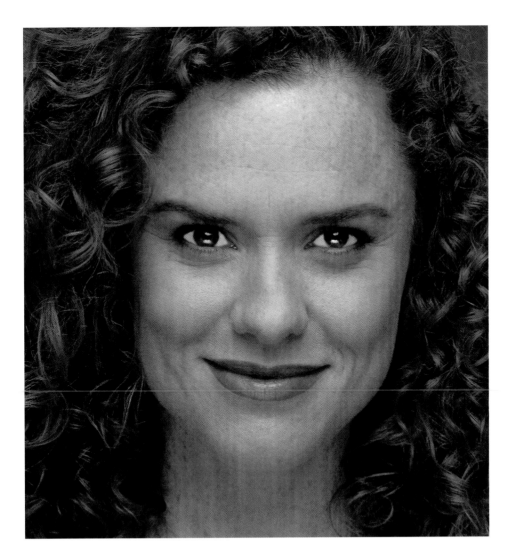

WIDE FACE For a face that holds a few extra pounds, blush can subtly create a slimmer look. I urge you to be confident that full cheeks actually look more youthful in real life, than the photogenic sunken cheeks of high fashion models. Again, it's all about the careful blend of light and dark shades to create the illusion of natural angles.

When applying, use darker blush in the "C" shape. Concentrate the color in the hollow of the cheeks, being careful not to place blush high on the temples. A lighter color on top of the cheekbones, under the darker color, and in the apple will slim the face.

FULL FACE TIPS:

- Concentrate your blush shades on the apple and high on the cheekbones.

- Keep the blush below your eyes.

- Applying color too close to your nose will cause your features to look crowded together.

- Dust your brush with brown eye shadow before dipping into the blush. While dark contouring powders will look artificial, the combination of two blush colors will simply create a darker overall blush.

- No stripes! Blend carefully or the illusion of slimming will disappear.

- A little light blush works well on the tip of your chin.

I have always had circles under my eyes—no matter how much sleep I get. I've tried concealers, aquapacks, you name it. Nothing helped. When I tried your suggestions of not wearing lower eyeliner and applying my blush not on top of my cheekbones, rather in the hollow, I was stunned. I could still see vague traces, but that's because I always look for them. When I stepped back from the mirror—THEY WERE GONE! Even my husband said my face looked brighter.

— E.B., New York, NY

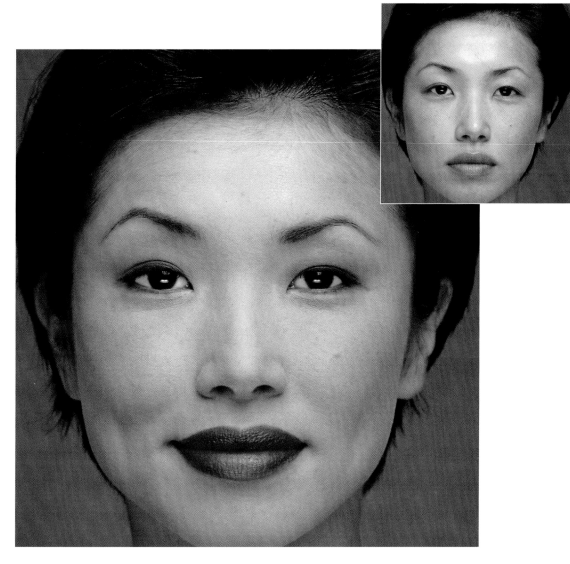

Whichever shape your face is, remember: Easy does it. The purpose of blush is not for contouring, although when used subtly, that may be the outcome. If a woman tries to create hollow cheeks or higher cheekbones, she'll inevitably be wearing too much. Her face will end up looking dirty or unhealthy, something we all want to avoid. In short, improperly blended blush applied with a heavy hand equals a makeup disaster.

That's one of the things a blush brush is for—to avoid war paint. If you've used too much, a sponge moistened with a little toner (water will cause bacteria to grow on the sponge) will absorb the excess color. A clean dry sponge used immediately afterward will help to reblend. If you remove too much, no problem. Just add more color.

CHOICES FOR RADIANCE

Do you recall the color you turned the last time you were embarrassed or excited? Or when you were exercising and felt that great rush of endorphins? Or even better, right when you finished making love? That's the color you're going for with your blush. If you've been in the sun and you have a light tan, your blush color will be different than in the dead of winter when your skin is completely pale. Choose your blush shades accordingly.

Selecting color can be a lot of fun. Start, as always, by gravitating toward the colors you like best. In order to try them on, apply a sample on your face over the foundation and powder you'll be wearing on a daily basis. Then, take a mirror into natural light to check the color. If your cheeks are so bright, they draw the attention away from your eyes, your blush is too dark. If the blush is lighter than your foundation, it's too light. It's not so complicated, is it?

I've found that pink blush is compatible with most eye makeup and lipsticks. Feel free to wear pink with peaches, corals, fuchsias, berry tones, and the brown-toned neutrals. Peach is another popular choice, but if there's too much brown in it, it will clash with blue-red or blue-pink lipstick or eye shadow. For women with dark complexions, pink blushes are often too light, and red is the best choice. Red works well for evening with any complexion, but always apply sparingly and blend with extra care. Personally, I avoid fuchsia and berry-toned blushes, as I think they look too harsh. Have you ever blushed fuchsia? Natural is the word to keep in mind, whichever shade you choose.

The correct use of blush, besides adding life and color to your appearance, is to define the inherent structure of your face, not to change it. Before you begin your application, make sure your foundation and powder are even and smooth. That will assure your blush going on evenly and make it longer lasting. Keep in mind that you want your blush to be blended with no demarcation lines and no harsh edges. Natural, natural, natural. Blend, blend, blend.

You may want to try different shades of blush for day and evening wear. I like softer shades in the daytime like beige or pink. When the sun goes down and I'm going to be in artificial light, I choose stronger, deeper tones, keeping in mind to match the lipstick I've chosen for that particular night. Using your lipstick as a blush match for the same color family is a trick that will usually steer you in the right direction, but there are exceptions to this rule. Sometimes we want to be bold and stray from what's

When your makeup arrived, my 15-year-old daughter and I watched your video, stopping to practice your techniques. Blending is really the trick! We were both thrilled at how flawless our skin looked.

— L.H. Paoli, PA

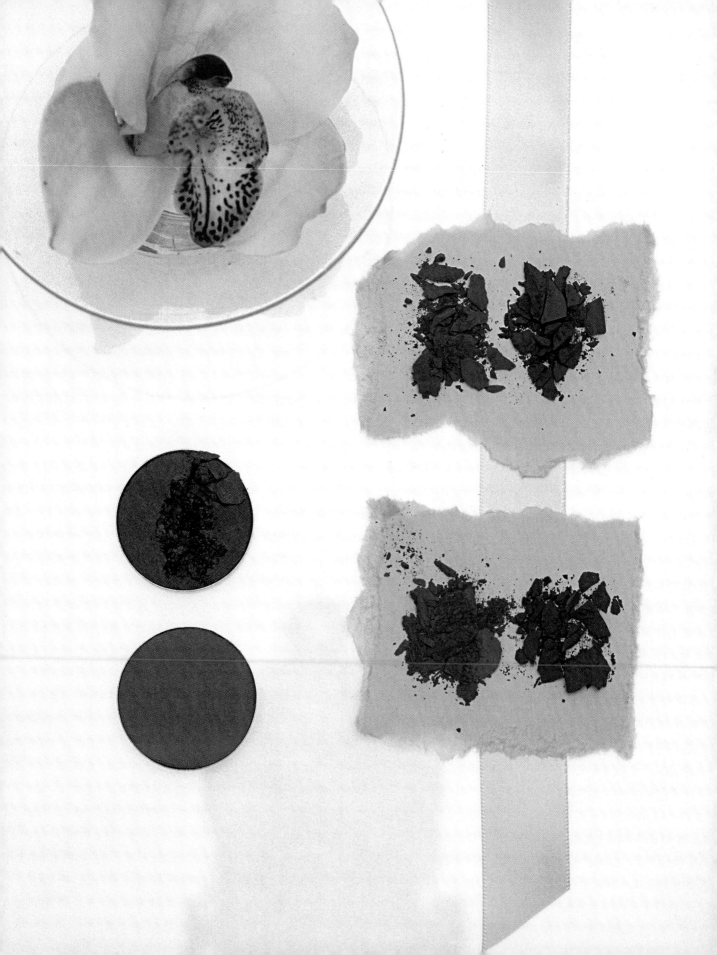

normally accepted. A good blend is what matters most, to make your face look balanced, and healthy.

Blush comes in several different forms:

- Cream blush has more natural richness and is sometimes a good choice for older women if their skin feels dry. A little powder lightly dusted over the top of the cream will increase its staying power. There are some wonderful shades available, but remember that cream tends to exaggerate imperfections in the skin.

- Gel blush is transparent and seems to be a good choice for teens. Since acne is often a teenage problem, I suggest you stay away from creams and stick with gels or powders. Keep in mind that blush will add to skin redness and accentuate imperfections.

- Powder blush, which is in my line, is the easiest to control. (Are you noticing a theme here?) It's also more forgiving. I like the easiest options, both for control and time-saving qualities, so choose according to your needs. The good news is that powder blush is longer lasting than the other options and a compact of blush has a shelf-life of up to two years.

Guidelines for choosing the right glow:

- Always try your blush on before buying it. Shades always look different in a compact than they do on your cheeks.

- A blush that's too light will look as artificial as one that's too dark.

- Vivid cheek color works best for a dramatic, evening look.

- Buy a light and dark color at the same time, making sure they blend together well.

- Save frosted or shimmery blush for special occasions.

BRONZERS A bronzer is especially useful when you have a tan or when you want to warm up your face. In these modern times, when getting a tan is bad for your skin, bronzers can provide an answer. There are several formulas available, so try them out and choose one that works best with your skin and the look you have in mind:

- Cream and stick bronzers are good for spot placement on cheekbones, nose, chin, and eyelids. Some women even use it on their lips. Stick and creams come in pinks, peaches, and browns. Anything overly orange tends to look unnatural.

To apply, lightly dab your sponge into the bronzer. Sweep onto cheeks and blend. You can also apply to forehead and chin if you wish. Correct with sponge and blend again.

- Powder bronzers are the quickest and easiest to use. I like them pressed but they also come in loose form. Powder bronzers can be used in winter as well as summer, because they tend to lay on less sheen than cream or stick. Shimmerless go on best, but you might like to experiment with shimmer from time to time.

  To apply, place a small amount on blush brush. Tap off the excess and brush cheeks, forehead, the crest of the nose and chin. Make corrections if you've overdone it.

GUIDELINES FOR BRONZER:

- Apply bronzer last, after foundation, powder, and blush or in place of blush.

- Bronzer is for adding color, not changing color.

- A loose powder bronzer, a half to one shade darker than natural skin will warm most skin tones. Pale faces generally don't take well to bronzers.

- A bronzer can stain the skin if not blended immediately.

- Cream and stick bronzers generally contain oil. For oily skin, to avoid breakouts, stick with powders.

BLUSH GUIDELINES:

- Lightly dust blush all over your face to add life and vitality.

- If you're not sure where to place your blush, just smile. It goes on the apple of your cheeks with a little bit beneath the cheekbone. Remember, no sculpting!

- If your blush goes on streaky, a little powder over your foundation first will help to smooth it out

- If you overdid your blush, no worries. Use your sponge to blend away excess.

- Avoid stripes of blush on your cheeks. It makes you look painted and unhealthy.

- Use lighter, more natural blush shades in the daytime. Darker shades work better at night. When in doubt, let your lipstick shade be your guide.

- A clean pale pink blush complements most complexions.

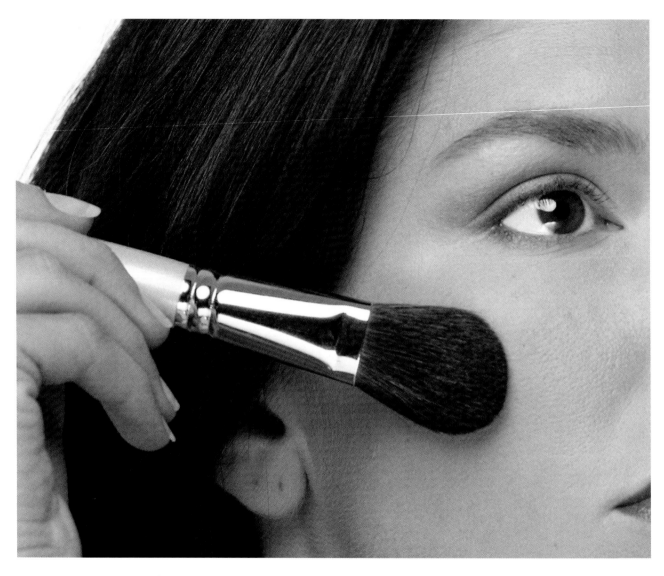

■ Pink with peach that is a few shades darker are good together for *lightly* defining the hollow of the cheeks. This combination works for most women from pale ivory skin tones to mid-tone dark brown.

■ For women with very dark complexions, a deeper pink on the apple with a red or intense pink or peach on the hollow may be your best bet.

■ For a quick pick-me-up, lightly dust the center of your eyelid with the lighter shade of my pink blusher. Feel free to use fingers for this quick eye-opener.

BEAUTY MARK
1:
A touch of blush toward the end of a long day will add a little color to your face and put some life back in your step.

BEAUTY MARK
2:
Blush is not a substitute for liposuction of the cheeks. Use it to add glow, not to create unnatural hollows.

BEAUTY MARK
3:
If you complete your eye makeup before moving to the cheeks, you won't mistakenly use too much blush.

BEAUTY MARK
4:
A little blush applied on lids, brow bone, nose, chin, and forehead will add radiance to the face. This will give you a sun-kissed look as these are the places the sun naturally hits.

BEAUTY MARK
5:
Bronzers used subtly and blended well can add warmth to the face, especially during the summer months.

APPLICATIONS *for* BLUSH

BLUSH—ACCENTING CHEEKBONES

Blush can act as a contour or high-light, or both, depending upon how it's applied.

1   Suck in cheeks, feel along cheek-bone tracing downward until you feel the natural hollow. This is where the darker color will be applied.

2   Using blush brush, apply darker color in deepest area, making a "C" shape from hollow, up to temple.

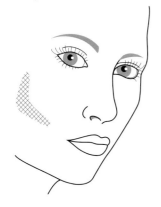

3   Smile, use lighter color lightly on apple of cheek.

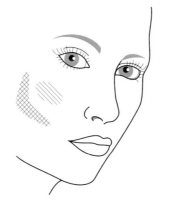

4   Blend lighter color on cheekbone into darker one.

5   Blush can be applied to nose, fore-head, and chin.

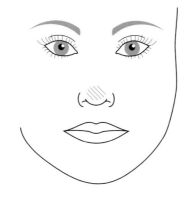

BLUSH FOR A LONG FACE

1   Suck in cheeks, feel along cheek-bone tracing downward until you feel the natural hollow. This is where the darker color will be applied.

2   With blush brush, apply darker color in hollow, making a "C" shape, blending up to temples on side of face.

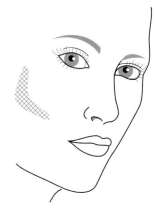

3 Use lighter shade blush on top of cheekbone, making sure not to work too high as to interfere with under-eye plane. This can make the eye look puffy.

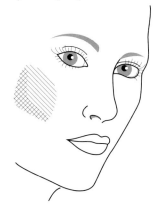

4 Smile, blend lighter color on apple of cheeks.

5 Try a little touch of blush on tip of nose for a sun-glow effect.

6 A light blushing of color on forehead and/or chin can help de-emphasize the length of face.

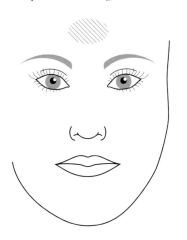

BLUSH FOR A WIDER FACE

1 Suck in cheeks, feel along cheekbone tracing downward until you feel the natural hollow. This is where the darker color will be applied.

2 With blush brush, apply darker color in hollow, making a "C" shape, blending softly up to outer side of eye.

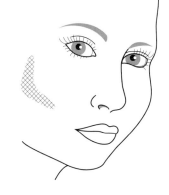

3 Do not blush higher than eye on side of face.

4 Use lighter color on top of cheekbone, blending it into darker shade.

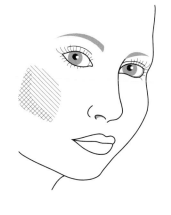

5 Use lighter color well below your darkest blush shade to aid in a slimming effect.

6 Smile, brush the apple of the cheek lightly with lighter shade.

7 Lightly brush tip of chin with lighter shade.

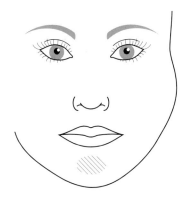

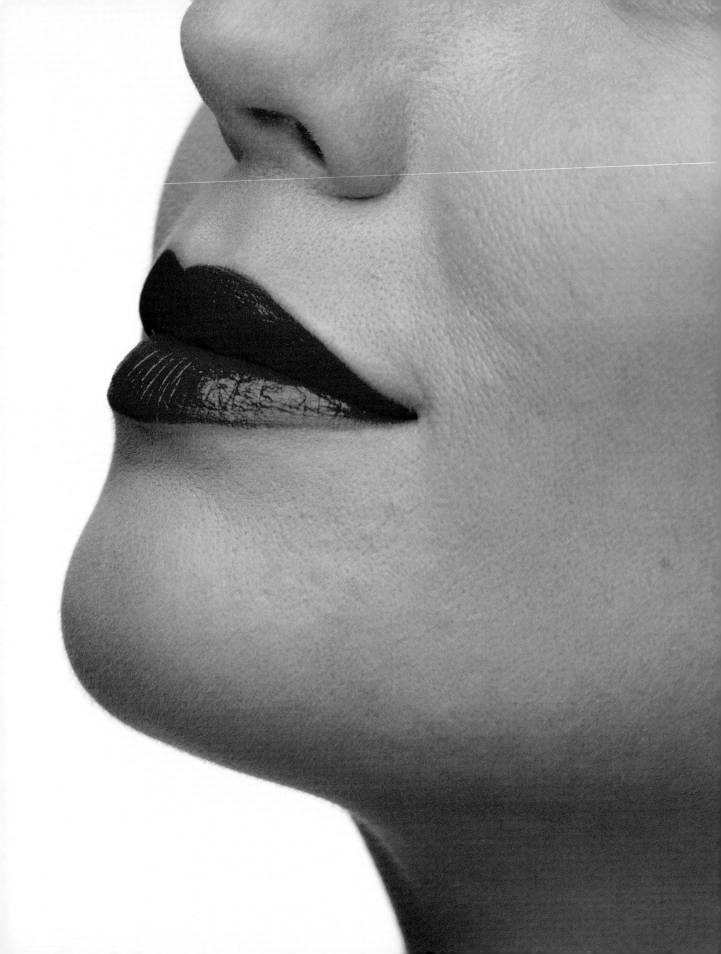

9: LIPS: FROM SUBDUED TO SENSUAL

PUMP IRON, NOT YOUR LIPS Can we have a serious discussion about lips here? Women are so busy these days trying to plump them up and fill them out and gloss them over and shape them into strange little peaks. Some women are even going to tattoo artists to have permanent lines drawn outside the natural contour of their own mouths—all to create what we've come to call a "succulent" mouth.

For me, a natural lip is the most appealing, and I expect we'll be returning there soon. In the meantime, if you jump on the bandwagon and have silicone or collagen injections, you'll end up looking like everyone else, instead of yourself, at best. At worst, your lips may end up looking artificial, disfigured, and you'll be out a chunk of change. Did you ever stop to think about what you'll do when the fad ends and delicate and demure is in again?

Whether you choose to create a more subdued look with a lip pencil, or you want to feature the lusciousness of your lips with strong color and gloss, fat, thin, or otherwise, lips are considered the most sensual feature on your face. In fact, they reflect your moods, so why pump them out, thin them down, or goop them up with tons of gloss? Just because Kim Basinger's lips are pouty, does that make pouty better for you? I'm not saying that gloss is unacceptable. It's great fun to play with lips, but it requires careful attention to what really looks good on *you* and what message you want to send.

MESSAGE IN A COMPACT
Lips say a great deal. I consider them to be the sensuous part of the canvas, where I want to use color and shape to draw attention. Have you ever noticed that when young girls play dress-up, they always go for the lipstick? That's because colored lips mean womanliness and they give off unmistakable messages.

Lipstick color is a definite form of self-expression, which is why I encourage women to blend their own shades. I put a variety of colors in each of my ten separate lip compacts, so you can build a lipstick wardrobe from there. You can create your color according to your complexion, how you feel that day, and the message you want to express. You may also want to change the message throughout the day, so it's nice to have options. When I feel as if my outfit isn't really alive enough, a nice vibrant lip color can somehow make it all come together.

Here will I dwell, for heaven be in these lips.
—Doctor Faustus,
by Christopher Marlowe

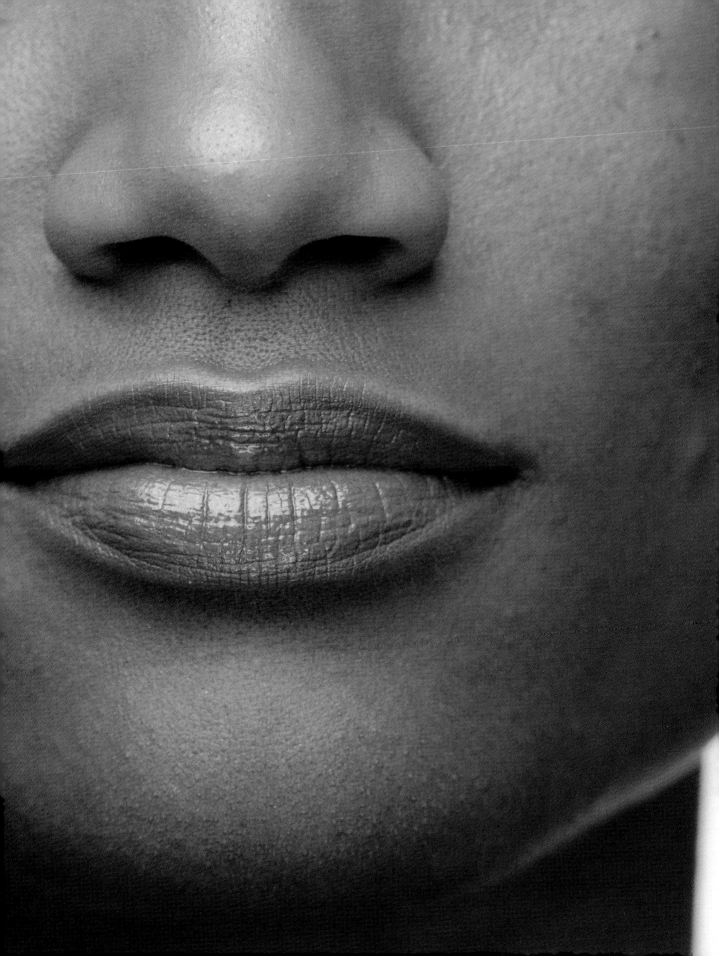

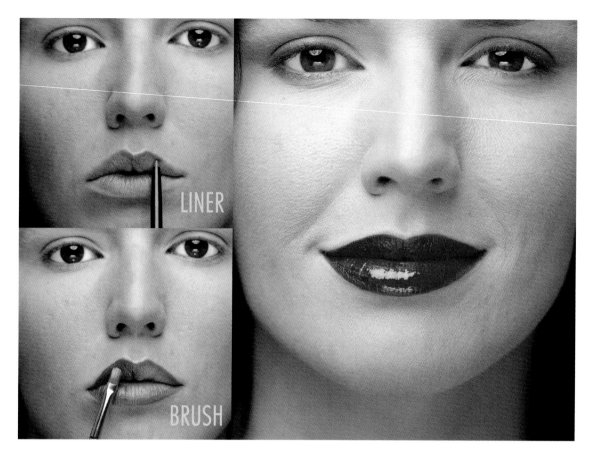

LINER

BRUSH

APPLYING LIPSTICK:

Here are my six steps for lipstick application:

- STEP #1: Always begin with dry, clean lips. Feel free to cover lips with foundation if your lipstick tends to wear off quickly.

- STEP #2: Define the bow of your lips with feathery strokes of your lip pencil.

- STEP #3: Define the line on each side of the bow with pencil. Start at top of bow and work toward outer corners.

- STEP #4: Line lower lip with pencil. Again, use feathery strokes.

- STEP #5: Fill in upper lip with color using lipstick brush or tube.

- STEP #6: Fill in lower lip with color on lipstick brush. Blot lips with a tissue. If you want longer-lasting results, use a pencil to cover entire lips, then apply color with brush, and blot with tissue.

Keep in mind: Open mouth slightly when applying lipstick, in order to stretch the lips taut. Puckering is out. Chapped, dry lips will not take color well. If chapping is your problem, lip balm can help. Avoid matte, long-lasting lipsticks, as they tend to dry out the skin.

A dab of gloss in the center of your finished lips, top and bottom, will look glamorous and create a fuller look.

STAY TRUE TO YOUR LIPS Lips shrink as we get older, and we need to accept that. Now don't panic and go running out to have them pumped up. Read on instead, because there are more creative ways to deal with this challenge. If your lips are less full than they used to be or if you have fine lines around your mouth, you can still create a compelling and sexy look. A common makeup mistake is to try penciling your lip line where it was when you were younger. This will look artificial, so give yourself a break.

We're back to seeing what you have and making the most or the least of it. A lip liner can help stop color from bleeding into the fine lines around your lips, but when it doesn't blend with your lipstick, it will draw attention to an area that you may not want to highlight. It's important to remember that no matter their size or shape. The ways in which you use your mouth to speak, smile, or show emotions (kissing falls into this category), all contribute to the distinctive beauty of your lips.

It follows that if your mouth is especially beautiful, emphasize it. If you think your eyes are the more striking feature, make up your mouth to be pretty, but not to be the focal point of attention. Keep in mind here that you can make minor adjustments with color that will create an illusion as to the size and shape of your lips.

TO LINE OR NOT TO LINE Lining the lips serves several purposes. First of all, it keeps your lipstick in place which is most important. Secondly, it defines the unique shape of your lips, something that makes you who you are. And finally, it helps you achieve special effects, such as minimizing or maximizing the size of your lips and still allowing them to look real and natural.

Lip liner is not as predominant in a makeup application as it used to be, so feel free to go without it if you have no special contouring goals. If you do, use liner wisely to create a look that pleases you, such as balancing unevenness, adding shape to lips that lack a bow, or solving aging problems like shrinking lips or fine lines. Always keep in mind that lip liner should blend, not stand out.

I use liner to keep color away from my fine lines and for definition. Lip pencils have become much softer which makes them easier to use. For more subdued lip color, pencils help.

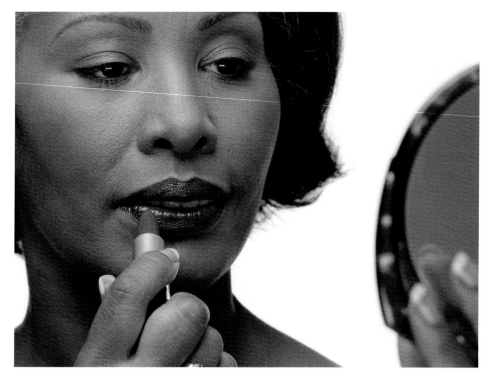

Even though I use a lip pencil (a slim one works best), and I blend my colors with a lipstick brush, it only takes me about thirty seconds to make up my lips. I could probably cut it down to ten seconds if I used a tube, instead, but I don't get the same precision. Practice, practice, practice, with your brush, and you'll find it's worth the extra ten seconds. Remember that you don't want your lips to compete with your eyes or vice versa. They need to work in balance so one enhances rather than one overpowering the other.

For more long-lasting lip color, after covering the entire lip with a pencil, add a coat of nonwaxy conditioner. This creates a natural-looking stain that will stay on your lips throughout a very long day and even into the evening. If you prefer tube lipstick, as some women do, don't neglect lining your lips with pencil.

Guidelines for lip liner:

- Apply liner in feathery strokes.

- For defining the bow of your lips, line the "V" with a lighter shade of pencil than you use for the rest. (Not too light.)

- For that desired pouty look, after applying lip color, add a lighter shade in the center of your lips.

- If your lips have an uneven tone, cover with foundation first, then proceed with application steps.

- For an unsteady hand when applying pencil, dip the fine edge of your wedge sponge into a bit of foundation and smooth along lip line.

Liner considerations:

- If your liner ends up too dark, your entire makeup will look wrong. Keep your mouth as natural-looking as possible when applying, even when the goal is to make minor adjustments. Lip liner should always appear subtle with no demarcation between liner and lipstick

- Age lines, although troublesome, won't diminish the beautiful shape of your lips. Avoid "supermoist" lipsticks which bleed into lines and accentuate fine wrinkles. If it doesn't dry you out, try using a matte lipstick after lining the lips with a pencil. Avoid lip glosses.

- Avoid drawing liner beyond the outside edge of your lips because the shape change will be too obvious. I call this "an overcorrected" lip. Allow the line to follow the outside edge of the ridge, and use a little extra foundation to highlight the bow. This will make your lips appear fuller, but not artificial.

WORKING LIP MAGIC There are so many ways to enhance your lips' natural shape and size, it feels like magic. Your mouth is defined by a ridge that covers the perimeter of the rosy lip pigment. I encourage you to use this ridge in determining the natural placement of color. In general, if you wish to minimize the size of your lips, line the inner edge of the ridge with a pencil and apply your lipstick right up to the liner, but not outside of it. For a fuller lip, line the outer edge of the ridge and extend your lipstick over the ridge to meet the liner. This way, you're following the natural line of your lips and achieving a contouring at the same time. Keep in mind that frosted or pale lipsticks tend to create the illusion of fullness, while a matte finish or more subdued colors do the opposite.

Magical contouring techniques:

- THIN LIPS: The secret to beautiful thin lips is to color them completely, without exaggerating the natural ridge line. As mentioned earlier, line the outside ridge and then fill in with color. This will create a wonderfully full look. To amplify color and keep the lips soft, a coat of nonwaxy lip conditioner will do the trick.

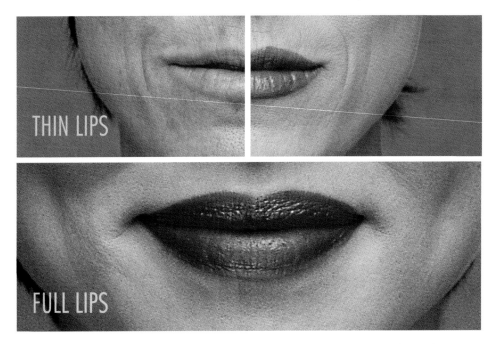

THIN LIPS

FULL LIPS

- FULL LIPS: The natural ridge serves as a beautiful frame for full lips. The secret here is to follow the contours of the lips inside the ridge for minimizing. If you wish to celebrate the fullness as it is, bring color to the outside of the ridge. Just go for it, you full-lipped women!

- UNDEFINED LIPS: With lips that are lacking the shape or fullness you want, you can strengthen with color and adjust the shape by a fraction. Begin by covering the center of your upper lip with foundation. If you need definition in the bow, draw a short, wide "V" in the center of upper lip. From the top of "V," extend the lines to the corners, rounding the curve of the bow. Line the outside edge of the lip ridge on your lower lip, fill in with color, and add a lighter shade in the center of your lips for highlights.

- UNBALANCED LIPS: Just because your lips aren't the same size, doesn't mean they're not beautiful, and I encourage you to leave them exactly as they are. If you wish to create a more balanced effect, line the outside edge of upper lip ridge, and follow the natural contours of your lower lip with no liner pencil. A slightly lighter lipstick on either lip will make it appear more prominent.

- DOWNTURNED MOUTH: If you want to make yourself look happier, extend the line of the upper lip *slightly* above the natural corner, creating a "<" and ">" on the skin. Then fill in lip color. To focus attention to center of lips, highlight the center only with a lighter shade of lipstick.

Guidelines for minor lip adjustments:

- If the natural pigment doesn't end up completely covered, use foundation.

- For the most natural look, round your bow peaks.

- To shorten wide lips, stop the lip liner within the natural corners.

- Never outline beyond the natural lip ridge. This will look artificial.

- To minimize lips, line the inner ridge. If you stop short of that ridge, the lips will look shapeless and unnaturally thin, which creates an angry expression.

LIPSTICKS: ALL TYPES
When you want to change your look, lip color is a good product to consider. Although they come in a variety of forms, all lip colors are basically made up of waxes, oils, and dyes. The most common types and their ingredients are:

- Creams are for the widest color selection and the smoothest application. Made from oils, polymers, pigment, wax, and vitamins, creams can produce a classic, rich, moist opaque mouth.

- Mattes are for long-lasting color, although they tend to be drying and more difficult to apply. Made from volatile silicones that instantly evaporate, leaving pigments and waxes, they produce a full, even no-shine coverage with colors that last for a long time. They've recently come out with a sheerer, moister form of matte, so check your stores.

- Satins are made from oils and polymers that lubricate the lips. They create a low-shine gleam, somewhere between a matte and a gloss, which creates a shiny finish.

- Stains are dyes that literally stain the lips, giving a dry finish that changes lip color. Sheer stains are also available for an even more fresh-looking stain.

- Transfer-resistant lipsticks are made from volatile silicones that vaporize fast and set the color. There's no smearing and the color lasts six to eight hours. If you've ever wondered how they do all that kissing in the movies and the man walks away without "lipstick on his collar," this is it.

- Lacquers are gel-based formulas available in pots, that deliver sheer color and leave you with a low-key shine.

- Semi-glosses are less gooey and shiny than regular gloss, which come in classic lipstick formulas rather than pots or wands.

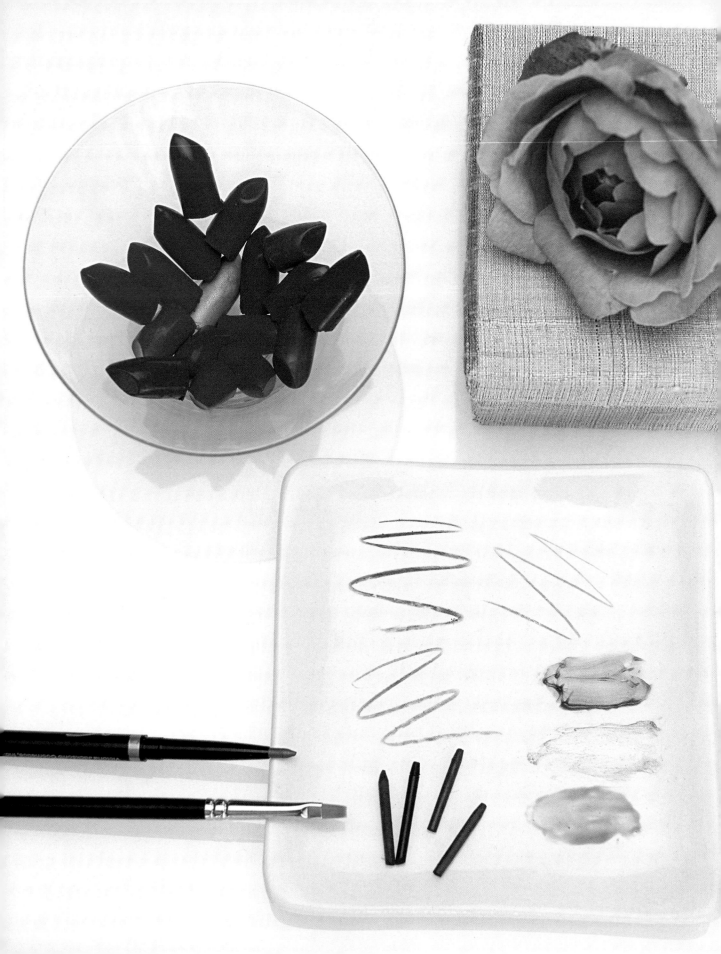

COLOR SELECTION I like cream lip compacts because of the wonderful texture, the ease in application, and the variety of choices to mix and match. This allows not only combining, but also changing color throughout the day. I group some of my shades in peach, pink, and red, and I like to use a lip brush for blending. This allows so many possibilities, and I can feel like an artist, choosing colors from my palette. Even though you'll probably gravitate toward a favorite color, be bold! Play with color and you may find some additional favorites you never considered. Sheer stains are good for summer, as they deposit less color. Matte textures give you a more polished look, while a little gloss can freshen you up.

A few summer hints:

- Giving your lips a matte finish is as easy as brushing one of the powder lipsticks from my Peach, Pink, or Red kits over your choice of lip color. This will give you a shimmery, silky finish that lasts. You can also set lip color by holding a single layer of facial tissue against your lips and applying powder with a brush over the tissue.

- For the most natural look of sheer color, after outlining and filling in with lip color, add lip conditioner over the top.

- For a soft, finished, luscious look, brush a layer of color over lips, blot, and then apply foundation sparingly around the outside edge of mouth with a triangular sponge. Once again, add more color but keep brush away from the edges of your mouth.

It's good to have a liner pencil that complements your lips or your lipstick. By the way, I've added lipstick tubes in my line because so many women requested them, but my four-color compacts still outsell the tubes. Remember that your lip brush should be flat and slightly tapered to glide around the curves of your mouth for precise color placement.

Many lip colors now contain sunblock which is a good way to go since the lips have so little protective melanin, they burn quickly. This is both painful and unhealthy, so if you ski or find yourself in the sun a great deal, this is very important to consider when buying lipstick.

A good way to choose color is to find a lipstick that looks good on your bare face. Then, the rest of your makeup will only enhance it. To help you with your decisions, here are some guidelines for selecting color for your lips:

- For sallow complexions, add a glow to your skin tone with bright shades of lipstick. Opt for the brownish shades if you like a more neutral lip. Oranges will only bring out yellow, so pass on these.

> *Make-up is a big part of my life because I spend so much time in front of the camera. I always find that a little gloss is nice to enhance my lips.*
>
> — *Vanna White*

- For ruddy complexions, peach or browns are best.

- For very fair complexions, a bluish cast will work well.

- For yellow teeth, (which happens as we age), avoid bluish shades. They'll only make your teeth appear more yellow.

- If you want to play it safe with color or you're just not sure, don't despair. A shade closest to the natural tone of your lips will always work.

Considerations for red lips:

- There are blue-reds, orange-reds, and brown-reds. One of these will work best for you, so take time to find the right one.

- To lighten red, mix red pencil with gloss and blot it down to the shade you prefer.

- Red pigment will actually leave stains on the lips, especially if you use them on a constant basis. Keep this in mind.

- Be careful if your face has redness or blotches. Deep red lips will draw attention to skin imperfections.

- Lip liner is a great help with red lipstick for perfect definition.

Tips to make color last:

- If your lipstick feathers, (comes off in small, intermittent sections), give your lips a primer before applying color. You can also lightly powder the lip ridges. Avoid glossy lip products.

- If the color seems to fade away, start with a little foundation. You can also fill in lips with pencil before applying cream, or color over them afterward. If you want to try several layers of lipstick, be sure to blot after each one. Matte formulas tend to stay on much longer, but they also dry out the lips.

- If your gloss seems to disappear, try a base of lip pencil first or a blotted down matte.

- If the liner tends to disappear, dip a cotton swab in lipstick to redefine the edges or use your trusty sponge to get rid of straying color.

Helpful Hints:

- If your lipstick tends to wear off quickly, cover lips with foundation.

- To calm down red, mix a red lip pencil with gloss to dilute the intensity of the shade.

- When applying lip liner, feathery strokes are more mistake-proof.

- To avoid lipstick on teeth, either blot with tissue or place your forefinger in your mouth, and after closing your mouth gently around it, withdraw finger. This will keep the rest of your lipstick intact.

BEAUTY MARK

1:

Keep your lipstick within your natural lip line. In other words, stay true to your lips.

BEAUTY MARK

2:

Keep your mouth in a natural shape while lining lips to help you find the natural lines.

BEAUTY MARK

3:

Don't get into a rut with color. Play and experiment, you'll be amazed at the different looks you can create.

APPLICATIONS *for* LIPS

TO RESHAPE THIN LIPS

1   Using lip pencil, draw above natural lip line, extending to outer rim of natural highlight. This will retain the natural shape of your lips.

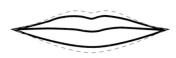

2   To shape lips, extend line further at bow and in center of lower lip, tapering to corners.

3   Apply lighter lip color.

TO THIN FULL LIPS

1   Cover upper and lower lip line with face foundation color.

2   Powder lightly to set foundation.

3   Line lips with lip pencil just inside natural lip line.

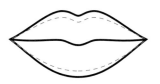

4   Apply lip color, keeping an even tone, so as not to add more shading.

TO EVEN OUT CROOKED LIPS

1   Cover fullest lip line or fullest lip line area with face foundation color.

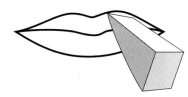

2   Powder lightly to set foundation.

3   Using lip pencil, line lips on full side just inside natural lip line.

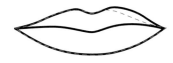

4   On thin side, line lips just outside natural lip line.

5   Be sure to balance lips and soften lines for a natural look.

6   Apply lip color.

FOR SHAPELESS LIPS OR TO SHAPE LIPS

1   To redefine lips, cover lip line with face foundation color.

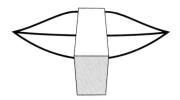

2   Powder lightly to set.

3   Using lip pencil, draw a "V" in the bow area of upper lip.

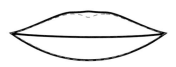

4   Extend line from each peak to corner of mouth. Slightly round peaks, so the "V" is not pointed. To strengthen top lip, add natural highlight line. Use lip brush and lightly follow just above your new lip line with lighter foundation color. Blend softly.

6   Apply lip color. Concentrate darker color in center of mouth and lighter in the corners.

TO SHORTEN WIDE LIPS

1 Cover corners of mouth with face foundation color using sponge.

2 Powder lightly to set foundation.

3 Using lip pencil, line lips stopping just short of mouth corners. Connect upper and lower lip line in mouth corners, slightly extending corners upward, so mouth does not appear to droop downward.

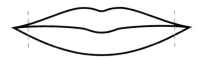

4 Strengthen natural highlight by drawing line with lighter foundation color, applying with the handle tip of lip brush. Lightly follow above lip line. Blend softly.

5 Apply color within lip line. Concentrate darker color in center of lips, working lighter in corners of mouth.

DOWNTURNED MOUTH

1 To turn a sad mouth into a happy mouth, extend lip line beyond mouth into skin and reshape corner with lip pencil. Make sure angle is slightly raised.

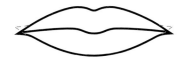

2 Continue lining lips, following natural lip line.

3 Apply lip color.

4 Remember to apply lighter lip colors to corner of mouth, keeping deeper shades in center.

TO EVEN OUT NATURAL LIP COLOR

1 If one lip varies in color from the other lip, cover both lips with face foundation using sponge. Lightly powder to set lips. Line lips with red pencil. Apply lip color with lip brush.

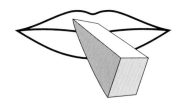

2 To strengthen natural highlight, line above lip, then using lip brush handle or cotton swab dip into lighter foundation color.

3 Following natural lip line, lightly apply foundation on natural highlight above lip. This should be applied very lightly. Blend.

115

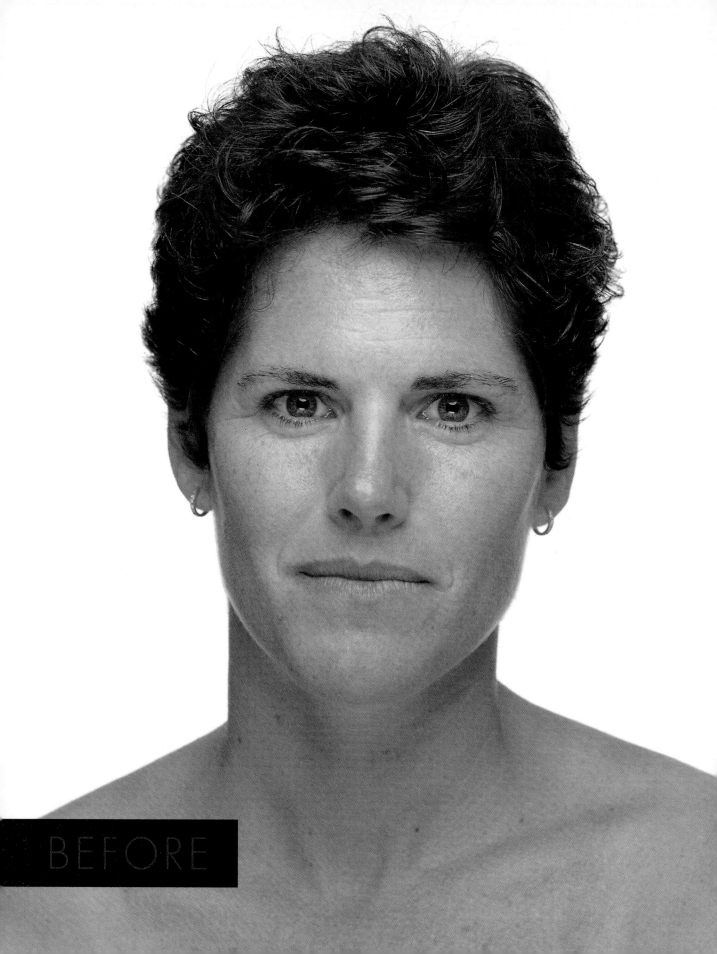

BEFORE

10: TWO-, FIVE-, & TEN-MINUTE FACE

CREATE THE FACE THAT SUITS YOU

Let's face it, women are all different, we move at different speeds, and we have different priorities. I know women who spend two minutes on their makeup in the morning, others who spend five on makeup for a television appearance, and still others who won't leave the house to shop without taking a good half hour for their faces.

If you're as busy as I am or if you're running late for an appointment, my two-minute face can make a significant difference in how you look, zoning in on what most needs enhancing so you'll feel confident. I have to admit that as much as I'd choose to spend more time on my makeup before a business

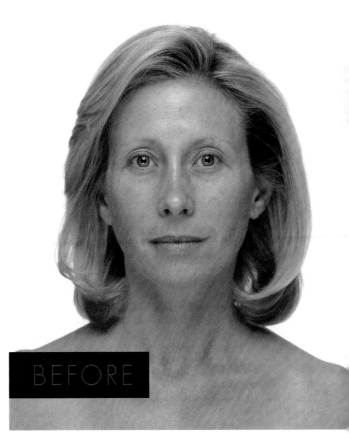

BEFORE

meeting, I've used this two-minute technique more than once, and it works! I'd also like to add here that twenty years ago, I felt better with two minutes for makeup than I do today in my forties, but in a pinch, it still works. People just seem to respond differently to me when I have on a little makeup.

When I have just a bit more time, I pay attention to my eyes by adding more shadow and mascara, still keeping the natural look in mind. This is when I take the five-minute approach. Special events or social occasions sometimes call for more makeup, so when I have a board meeting or I'm going out for dinner, I appreciate taking a few minutes extra to feel special. I always want to look like myself, but I also want other people to focus on my eyes. The little extra effort, if I can find the time, is always worth it.

If we accept the fact that we look beautiful with no makeup at all, we can choose how much energy we want to devote to our faces, according to available time and interest. If you love applying makeup, you'll probably take greater care with it. If you don't, you'll become a two-minute master. I rarely spend more than ten minutes on my face, even for a special event, but for me, it's enough. The truth is, if you learn to apply makeup correctly, ten minutes will be plenty of time to bring out your natural radiance. If you feel like lolling in front of the mirror for a while and you have the time, be my guest!

THE BASIC TWO-MINUTE FACE
My two-minute face is a minimalist approach. It's my emergency door, and I find it convenient, efficient, and best of all, effective. In essence, I can put on some foundation, highlight my eyes and cheeks, play up my lips a little, and still get the kids to school on time. Sure, I can run out the door with no makeup at all (that does happen from time to time), but I've noticed the extra two minutes on my face also seems to give me an extra edge of self-confidence. I suppose being in the beauty business makes me more focused on it, but you just may discover that it works for you, too.

For my two-minute face, vary the following instructions to suit your particular needs. I've included the basic formula with a couple of variations.

■ FOUNDATION — FORTY-FIVE SECONDS.
Apply foundation sheerly all over your face, including eyelids. Use a clean sponge to blend again and absorb the excess.

■ BROWS — TEN SECONDS
A few strokes of brow pencil will strengthen your eyebrows and frame your face.

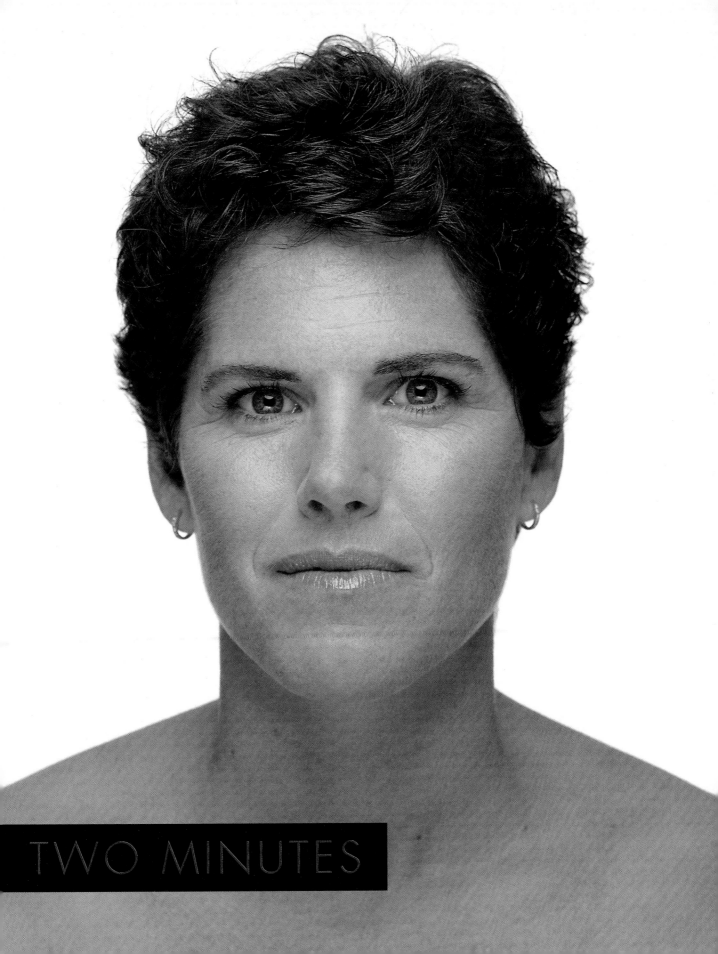

TWO MINUTES

- ▨ EYE SHADOW – FIVE SECONDS

  With a light touch of eye shadow, your eyes will come alive and any discolorations will disappear.

- ▨ EYELINER – TWENTY SECONDS

  Use the taupe eyeliner pencil on top and bottom lids. Smudge line to a soft shadow.

- ▨ MASCARA – TEN SECONDS

  Roll one coat on top and bottom lashes.

- ▨ BLUSH – TWENTY SECONDS

  Lightly dust apple of cheekbones with a natural blush shade of your choice.

- ▨ LIPS – TWENTY SECONDS

  To put on color that will last, line and fill in lips with pencil that blends well with your blush.

TWO-MINUTE VARIATIONS

If you want to concentrate on your eyes, spend only thirty seconds on spot foundation, then use thirty seconds for brows, thirty-five for shadow, liner, and mascara. Ten seconds for a hint of blush will leave fifteen seconds for lips.

Or:

Spend forty seconds on a total foundation. Don't forget to blend. Line and smudge eyes for about twenty seconds. Shadow takes ten seconds, while blush is done in fifteen seconds. For a nice lip finish, line and fill in with pencil for twenty seconds. Use ten seconds to add blush touches on nose and chin, and have five seconds to take a sip of coffee!

HELPFUL HINTS FOR THE TWO-MINUTE FACE:

- ▨ If you have dark eyebrows, the mascara that's left on your wand when you complete your eyes, is an adequate brow cover.

- ▨ Keep your two-minute tools in one place on your nightstand or in the bathroom. Who wants to waste precious seconds searching for makeup?

- ▨ Whenever possible, spot foundation rather than doing a full cover. It gives you a few extra seconds for other areas.

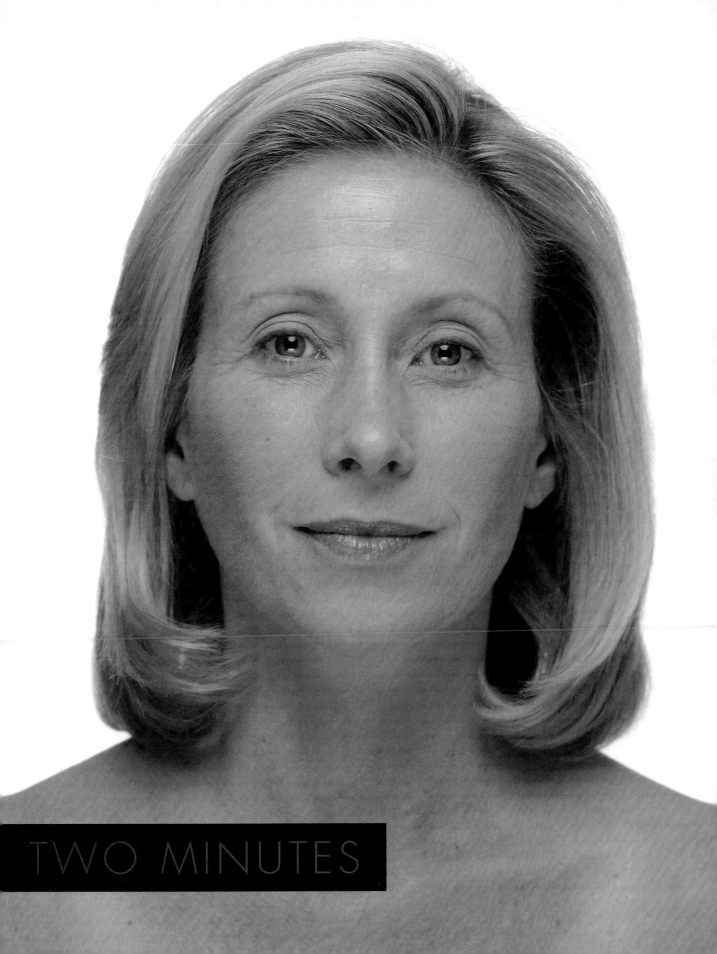

TWO MINUTES

THE BASIC FIVE-MINUTE FACE

Five minutes may not sound like much, but compared to two minutes, you can achieve some wonderful makeup effects. With the three extra minutes to spend, a five-minute face will allow you to look a little bit more pulled together. Some added attention to each of your features will make a difference, because you can be more picky.

You'll see that this approach is simple, building upon the two-minute face.

- **FOUNDATION – SIXTY SECONDS**
  With the extra time on foundation, you can cover your whole face.

- **BROWS – FORTY SECONDS**
  Make your brows really come to life with your brow pencil. There's more time to pay attention to shaping and definition.

- **EYE SHADOW – SIXTY SECONDS**
  Use the right color shadows to enhance the eyes even more.

- **EYELINER – SIXTY SECONDS**
  Take the time to line your eyes following the instructions in Chapter 7.

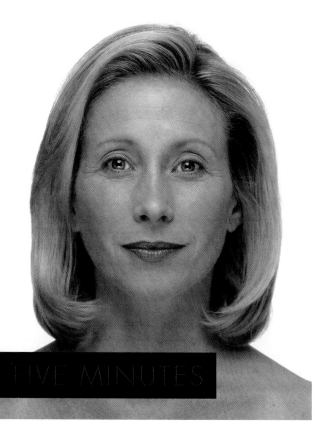

- **MASCARA – TWENTY SECONDS**
  What a luxury! Use the extra ten seconds to comb through lashes to separate clumps.

- **BLUSH – THIRTY SECONDS**
  After dusting the apple, you can also sweep a small amount of another color below cheekbones to add depth.

- **LIPS – THIRTY SECONDS**
  Use pencil for lining and filling in color.

FIVE-MINUTE VARIATIONS

If you need to minimize under-eye shadows and any discolorations around nose or mouth, take a full sixty seconds on your foundation, practically an eternity. Allot thirty seconds for your brows, and take a minute for liner, a minute to sweep on a couple shades of blush, and another minute for mascara. That leaves thirty seconds to devote to coloring and lining your lips, just enough time for some color mixing.

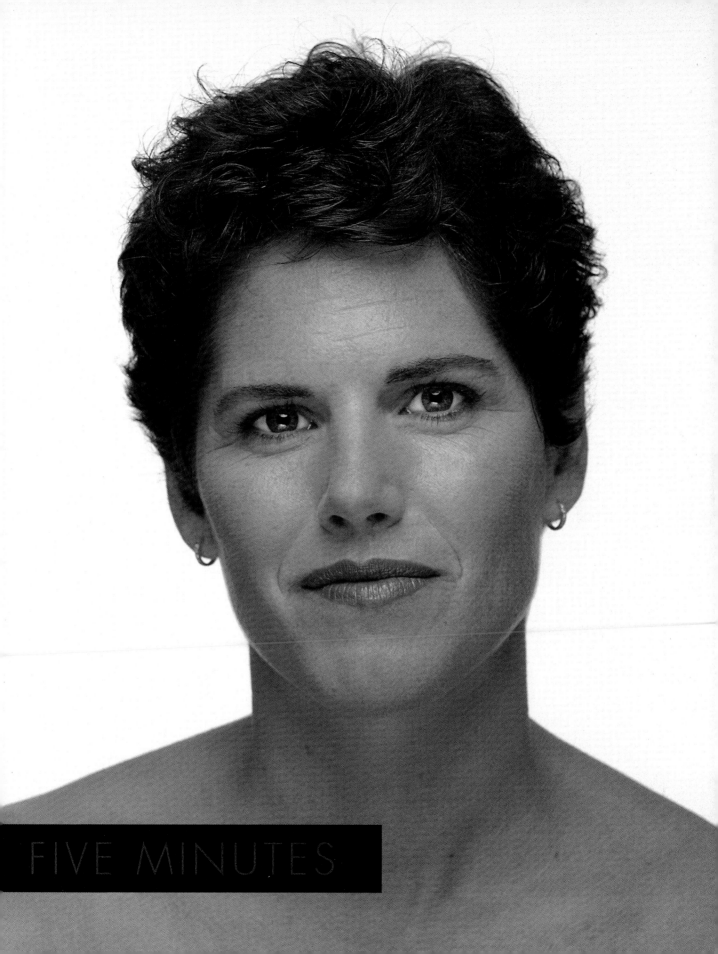

FIVE MINUTES

Another possibility—Use forty seconds for foundation. Then spend two full minutes on the eyes to blend two colors of shadow and liner. Mascara uses up twenty seconds, take a minute for blush, and use the last minute to line lips and fill in with real lip color.

HELPFUL HINTS FOR THE FIVE-MINUTE FACE:

- Start with your basic two-minute face and enhance!

- Five minutes will take the two minutes to a less sporty look.

- Have confidence that five minutes is enough—because it is.

- The five-minute face will work for both day and evening.

THE BASIC TEN-MINUTE FACE In ten minutes, you can create a glamorous image. The key here is to keep blending and layering so you don't look overdone when you're finished.

- FOUNDATION — TWO AND A HALF MINUTES
Apply a sheer foundation evenly and take the time to blend well. Even if you're using two shades for subtle contouring and dusting with powder, 150 seconds will give you ample time.

- BROWS — NINETY SECONDS
A soft pencil used carefully will define and enhance eyebrows.

- EYE SHADOW — NINETY SECONDS
Look into the specks of your irises and use two shades that bring out the best in your eyes. Blend well. You have time.

- EYELINER — NINETY SECONDS
Line your eyes with pencil, getting as close as possible to the lash line. There's adequate time to do top and bottom.

- MASCARA — FORTY SECONDS
Easy does it. Apply several coats if you wish and remember to comb well to remove clumps.

- BLUSH — FORTY SECONDS
Color the apple, subtly contour beneath the cheekbone and blend well with sponge. Stop and look for a few seconds and make sure you have on the right amount of blush for your face. At the end, you can check again so go light.

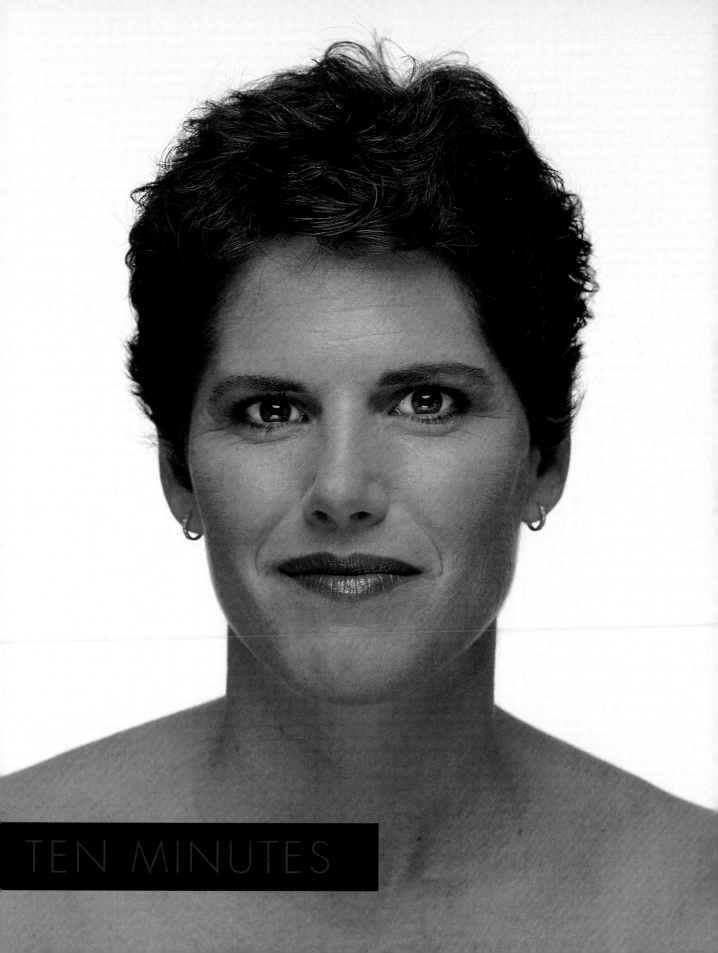

TEN MINUTES

■ LIPS — FORTY SECONDS

Line your lips with feathery strokes, then mix a fabulous color that makes you happy for filling in your lips.

Use the remaining minute to take an overall look at the end and make corrections.

TEN-MINUTE VARIATIONS
You can look very sophisticated by using two shades of blush to emphasize your cheeks. In order to blend carefully enough to avoid that "war-paint" look, allow two minutes for blush. With ninety seconds for foundation, darken your brows a little bit more, that'll take about ninety seconds.

Intensify eye shadow for ninety seconds, and allow another two and a half minutes for mascara and eyeliner. Don't forget to smudge! Allot two full minutes for lining lips with red pencil and coloring with red lipstick. Take the remaining thirty seconds to admire yourself!

Or:

For greater eye definition, try using liquid eyeliner on your top lids and pencil on the bottom. Smudge the bottom well, but leave the top alone. That'll take about two minutes, and your eyes will look larger and more dramatic. Allow two minutes for foundation, then blend two shades of blush for ninety seconds. Spend a minute on two coats of mascara. Deep shades of red lip liner and red lipstick will add on about two minutes. Now you can go anywhere!

HELPFUL HINTS FOR THE TEN-MINUTE FACE:

■ Just because you have extra time, don't overdo it. You still want to look like you.

■ If you've really brought out your eyes, go for a subtler lip color. Balance is everything!

■ If you use extra blush, blend to avoid the "war paint" look.

■ Liquid eyeliner can create dramatic eyes, but take time to apply carefully, since it's difficult to correct.

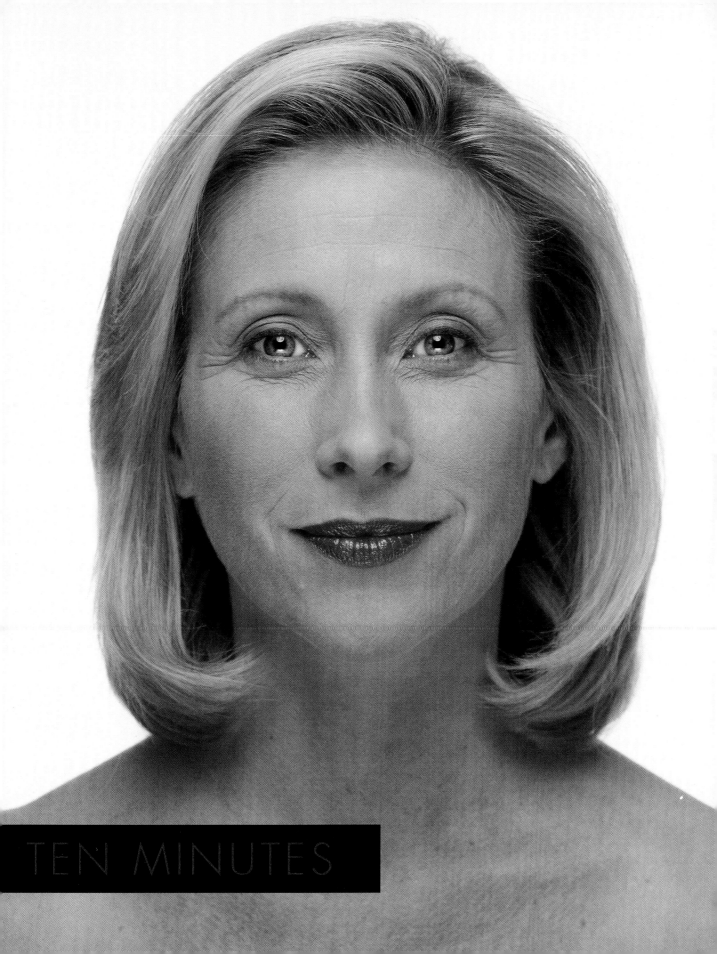

TEN MINUTES

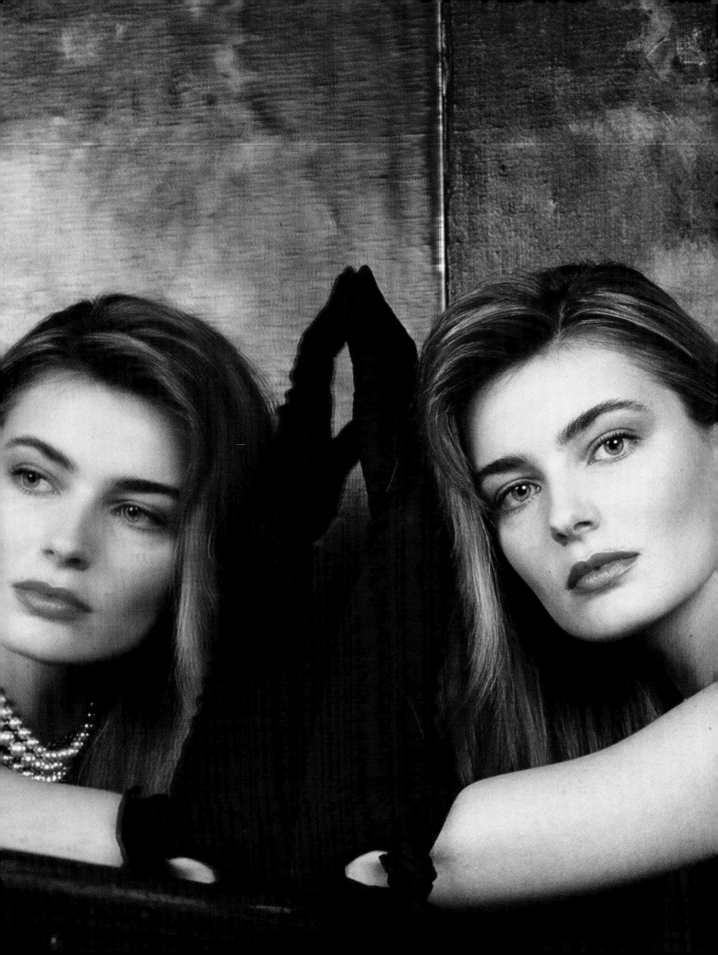

11: FROM DAWN TO DUSK: MAKEUP & HAIR TIPS

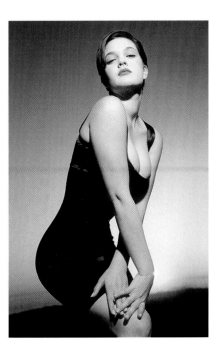

DO YOU KNOW WHERE YOUR HANDS ARE?

No matter what time they start out in the morning, many women need their makeup and hair to last all day long and often well into the night. Of course, if you can, you'll want to do a quick touch-up from time to time during those extended hours, but what if you can't? These days, many of you don't even have the time to run into a bathroom to check your faces (I know I sometimes don't), so redoing between appointments can be pretty much a fantasy.

I've heard women say, "By the time I get to the office or leave for lunch, it's as if I never put on my makeup. Why did I waste all that time in front of the mirror?"

Where does makeup go? Does it simply disappear? I don't think so. There are a few basic ways to keep your makeup from abandoning you and your hair from falling flat. One is to keep your hands off your face and out of your hair during the day. Ask yourself throughout the day, "Do I know where my hands are?" If your makeup seems to be smearing off for no apparent reason, you'll be amazed at the unconscious behavior patterns you've probably picked up. Do you stroke your cheeks to help you think? Do you rub your eyes when you feel weary? Do you put your hand against your lips when you're holding your tongue about something? Do you twist your hair in ringlets to help you make decisions? All these things will smear off your makeup and mess up your hair.

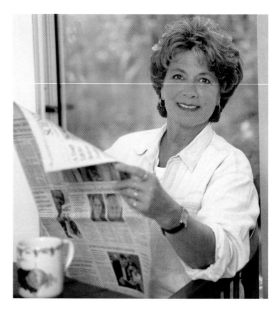

The telephone is another makeup dissolving culprit. Do you place the phone against your cheek when you're talking? A headphone is a big help if you have to be on the phone all day. It'll help keep your shoulders and your spine in alignment, too.

The biggest contributors to your makeup's dissolving into thin air are the quality of your cosmetics, how suitable they are for your particular skin, and the condition of your complexion. If your skin tends toward the oily side, be sure to seal in your foundation with powder. Pay attention to the type of moisturizers you use and how much you're putting on your skin. Oil-based ones will tend to create smearing of your makeup, so be careful. Nonoily moisturizers like the one I created for my line will allow your natural glow to show through, while controlling the oily content of your skin.

If you're a working woman, and you're going out at the end of a long day, you need to know what makeup tools to pack in the morning. This is why I created my survival kit. Using my own life as the template, I tried to put together everything I needed during the busiest day of the year.

Whether you're out on the run for the afternoon or you need to transition into evening, I've

> *I have three children and I baby-sit for four others. I put on my makeup each day at 5:30 A.M. and during the rest of the day I don't have time to even look in the mirror. I had a doctor's appointment last week at 6 P.M. and the first thing the doctor said was, "You look so fresh, like you just got out of the shower." That was all I needed. I was exhausted, but you can imagine how that made me feel after not having touched-up my face since before dawn.*
>
> *—J. F. Rocky Point, NY*

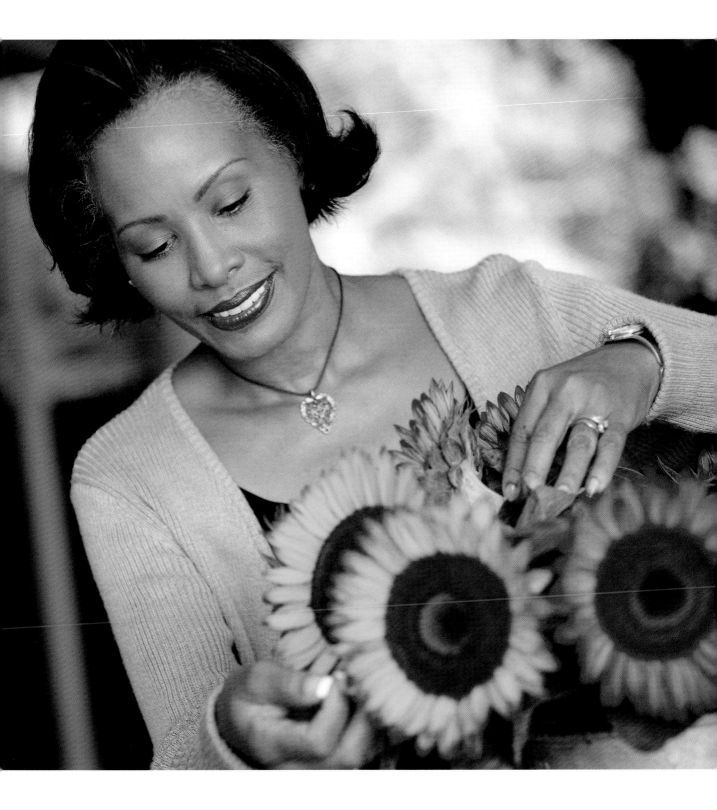

gathered the most important, multipurpose items I could find for any day and any look you may need to create. This kit contains two mirrors, an eye pencil that can double as a brow pencil, five separate shades of eye shadow and an applicator, mascara, two shades of blush with a blush brush, ten wonderful lip colors, and a lip brush for easy application. Besides a foundation compact which you'll have to carry separately, what else could a woman need? If you're a woman who works eighteen-hour days, I hope they find a way to change that. In the meantime, I'm proud that my survival kit can get you through some grueling times. I like the fact that it's small enough to fit into your purse, but whether you use my kit or something else, the idea is to have all the things with you that you may need throughout the day. When you need a pick-me-up, you can duck into a washroom for quick touch-ups and a few refreshing color changes with your blush and lipstick.

MIXING AND MATCHING
COLORS IN A PINCH
When I first did my color concept for TV, I introduced the news that one of the secrets of easy and quick touch-ups is to use colors in the same family. Then I manufactured three different color kits in peach, pink, and red, in which all the eye shadows, blushes, and lipsticks complemented each other and worked on almost every skin tone.

I can't tell you how many well-meaning intruders tried to discourage me from my idea. "People won't buy makeup if they can't see the colors," they warned me. "You're crazy to choose colors for them because they don't know how to picture them." I'm so glad I didn't listen, because, boy, were they wrong! The idea of a predetermined color kit was exactly what women were yearning for.

With a precoordinated color kit, if you need to dash into the restroom somewhere to freshen up your face, you won't be concerned as to what goes with what. The beauty of my concept was that you could take the blush from the red kit, for example, and it

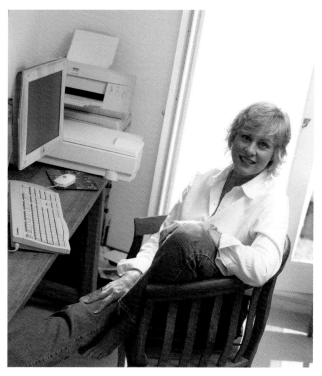

would look terrific with the lipstick in the peach kit. That results in endless makeup possibilities and endless fun. Feel free to play and experiment. In a pinch, though, when there's no time or room for error, you can use one kit by itself. What security to have when you're in a hurry.

I named my combinations "morning, noon, and night" for obvious reasons. The morning kit contains soft, pretty shades that work well in soft, early light, the noon kit is a little more intense for overhead sunlight, while the evening colors are vibrant and dramatic for artificial light or the dusty, romantic hues of evening. In the spirit of my experimental philosophy, you can interchange any of them as you wish, but again, if you need to do quick applications during the day, they're each arranged to match perfectly. Sometimes, even the most creative among us like to eliminate makeup choices when there are more important life decisions to face.

ALL ABOUT HAIR Most people don't know that my earliest beauty training involved becoming a hair dresser. In order to get my cosmetology license, I had to complete sixteen-hundred hours (that was roughly ten months), learning all about hair—cutting, coloring, perming, and styling. You name it, I did it. Although my real passion lay in makeup, I had some great experiences during my reign as a hair and makeup artist. Fairly early in my career, during a photo shoot for Ringo Starr's album cover, I had the opportunity to cut his hair. Many celebrities' haircuts followed, often in my home, where the locks of the rich and famous were strewn across my kitchen floor.

In the same way that your eyebrows frame your eyes, so your hair frames your whole face. My preference for hair is generally soft, pretty, and feminine. Whatever your preference, my advice is to make sure you walk out of the beauty salon with a hairstyle that works for *you*, not only your hairdresser or your friend who came along for the ride. I encourage you to speak up and not allow your stylist to dictate the way your hair should look. Remember that he or she won't be there to style it before you start your day, so make sure your hair is manageable—for you!

I start my day by evaluating where I'm about to go and how long I have to look my best without a touch-up. That varies, depending on my appointments for the day and whether or not I'm going to work out. Some days, I know I can tie my hair back and look just fine. Other mornings, I need to style a little bit more aggressively, and use hair spray to get me through.

In the afternoons, I do a quick brush through, if I can. If not, what you see is what you get. If I have an important meeting in the afternoon, I make time to reassess the hair situation and make sure that it works. It's the same idea as doing your makeup to put it behind you. You don't want to be worrying about your hair instead of closing a big deal.

We're lucky that big hair in the evening is a thing of the past. Today, we can get dressed to the nines and still have our hair casual and pretty. It's fun to experiment with your hair for an evening event, but it's also great to know you can pull it together quickly and still look terrific.

When it comes to hair color, consider your skin tone. Contrast between your skin tone and hair color will help your overall makeup application to enhance your best features. To help your colorist determine the right shades for you, wear your usual makeup so you can both get a sense of the finished look.

Remember—Choose your weapons wisely. Either your makeup or your hair should make the dramatic statement. Not both.

A FEW WORDS ABOUT LIGHT

Do your first makeup of the day according to the light you're about to be seen in. This is important because light reflects, and overdone makeup will be obvious. Since light changes throughout the day, making up for natural light will be your best bet. Then, if you find time to per-

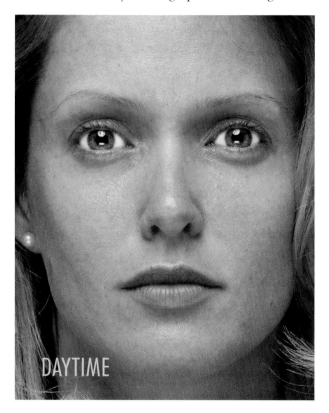

DAYTIME

form touch-ups throughout the day, they can be minimal.

If you're lucky enough to have natural light where you do your makeup, good for you! If not, keep in mind that most commercial makeup lights tend to be warm and yellow, so you may need to compensate. Try buying daylight bulbs that are bluer in tone. They're cooler, but they give off a cleaner cast. When you're buying makeup in a department store, the cosmetic counters use pink lighting which tends to cast a lovely glow on aging skin. The problem is that it tends to make your complexion look better than it is, so don't be fooled. As soon as you get into the real world, the light won't be so forgiving. When you try on makeup, take a mirror and walk outside into natural light to see the true shades. You'll be surprised at how different they look!

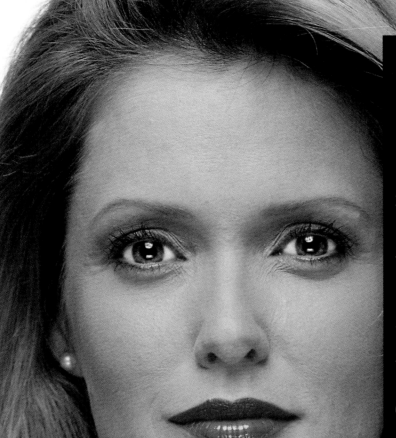

1 *Strengthen eye shadow, a little darker at outer corner and on eyebrow bone.*

2 *Add a touch of iridescence, if desired.*

3 *Line under bottom eye lashes with brown or black pencil. Smudge with cotton swab for a smoky look.*

4 *Add extra coat of mascara.*

5 *Add a touch of shimmer to your lips.*

6 *Strengthen lower lip pout by using a darker lip pencil in center below lower lip line.*

EVENING

If you're in a store in a large mall and going outside is impossible right then, try taking some swatches away with you. When I can't test something on my skin because I don't want to mess up my current makeup, the tester is not sanitary, or there's no available light that feels true, I take a piece of white paper or white tissue and do what people in the makeup business call "a draw down." It's a color smear with a Q-tip from particular shades that interest me. Then I take them outside later and examine them in sunlight. When you look at a lipstick in the store, all you see are the top tones. It's amazing how different a shade of red can look when you can clearly see all the undertones. It might be more purple, blue, or brown. I can't tell you how much money this process has saved me!

HELPFUL HINTS:

- Always know where your hands are—not on your face, I hope.

- Keep your skin well-conditioned. This helps your makeup last longer than most people realize.

- Color combinations in the same color family will save time for touch-ups by removing guesswork.

- Refreshing your lipstick can make it appear as if you've put on a whole new face of makeup.

- Light reflects, so take it into consideration during makeup applications.

BEAUTY MARK

1:

Make the dramatic statement with either your makeup or your hair.
Not both at the same time.

BEAUTY MARK

2:

Wear your usual makeup when determining the right hair color.

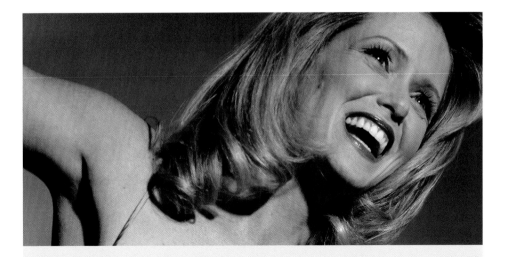

MYTH:

YOUR "SEASON" DETERMINES THE APPROPRIATE COSMETIC CHOICES.

REALITY:

DON'T BE LIMITED BY SYSTEMS THAT WERE CREATED BY SOMEONE
WHO DOESN'T KNOW YOU.

I've seen over and over again, that every woman can wear any color she likes at certain times. Why be limited by a system created by someone else, who has never even seen you? Why believe that a redhead can't wear red? I've seen some fabulous redheads looking smashing in burgundy dresses with rose-colored lipstick. I've also seen brunettes wearing purple or olive green and totally catching people's eyes, even though the "season experts" may have cautioned her against these colors.

There are varying shades of all colors that will flatter anyone, no matter your hair or eye color, according to the flecks of color in your irises that you may never have been aware of. It takes some investigation and experimentation to find what works best, but it's worth it. The only color rules I like to follow are that foundation shades lighter than your natural complexion generally don't look great, and coordinating the colors you choose will give you the best results. Beyond that, the world is your palette. Makeup is for creativity and expansion, not rigidity and limitation, so be an artist. Mix, match, and play. You'll be delighted in your finished product.

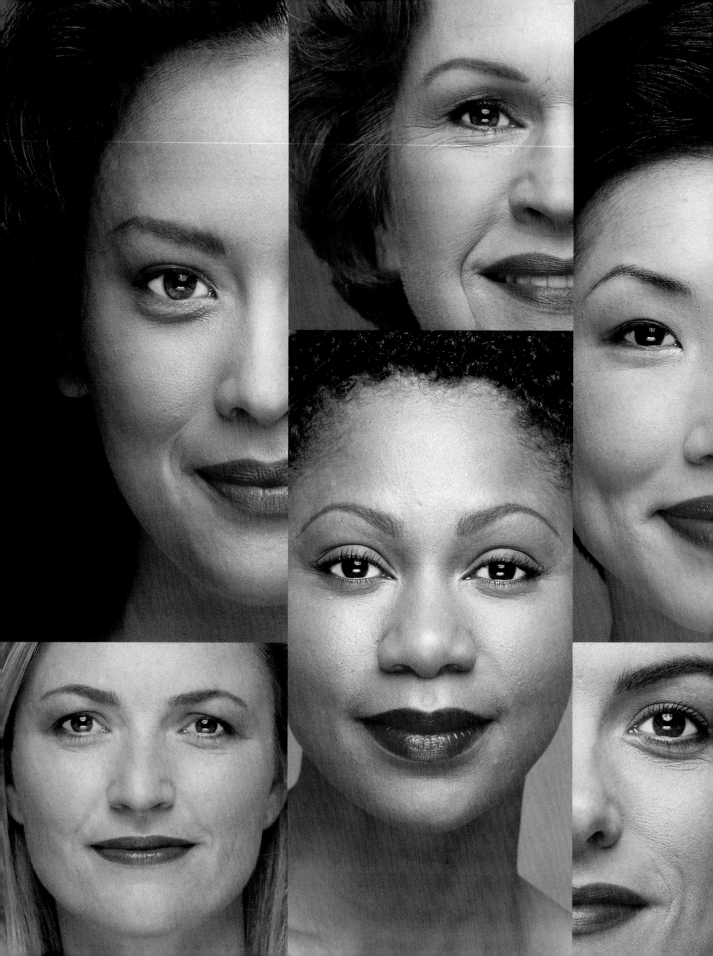

12: CELEBRATING DIVERSITY

KEEP YOUR MIND OPEN When I was a makeup artist, before I started my cosmetics company, I saw a great deal of racial stereotyping. Women of color believed they could only wear particular shades of lipsticks and blushes, and only one or two foundation colors. Most of them weren't trying new approaches, they were just accepting the limitations of the time.

I just couldn't buy it. I began experimenting. I couldn't see any reason why the makeup colors I used for a Caucasian woman wouldn't work on a woman of color. I went for it and the results were wonderful! Diversity became an integral part of my intention when I created my line of Victoria Jackson cosmetics. I not only wanted the best quality and a great variety of choices, but I wanted my colors to work on everybody and on all skin tones.

Shari Belafonte, a very attractive African-American woman actress with a relatively light skin tone, was one of the exceptions to the rule. When I first saw her, I complimented her on how great her makeup looked. When I asked how she'd avoided being close-minded, she said she was simply not interested in any kind of stereotypical thinking. She believed that women of color could and should be able to use any colors they chose. We were happy to find each other because we shared the same philosophy. We had some wonderful conversations about makeup and how we wanted to see other women playing with color as she did.

"Someone just needs to tell them it's okay," she said with a big smile. I was ready to accept her challenge. I've been encouraging all women to play with makeup ever since. Common sense will dictate what works and what doesn't. I wouldn't suggest a very dark-skinned woman to use my taupe eyebrow pencil, it simply won't show up and the color will be lost. That makes sense, just as a blonde woman with porcelain skin wouldn't use a dark brown foundation. It would look ridiculous, not because blondes aren't allowed, but because it wouldn't make her look her best.

America has become such a melting pot for exquisitely beautiful women of all colors and creeds, we hardly differentiate any more. I encourage women from around the world, no matter their race, simply to think of themselves as beautiful, exotic creatures and make their beauty choices from that point of view. I don't care if you're Asian, African-American, Hispanic, Caucasian, or Native American, a bad hair day is bad hair day. Who looks in the mirror on a day she isn't feeling well and says, "If only I were a different race, then I'd be beautiful." Rather, we try to figure out what to do with what we've got. If you celebrated a little too hard the night before, your eyes will look puffy whether you're from Sudan or Stockholm, and you'll need to make the proper makeup adjustments.

Keep in mind on those days when you feel bad and you think you look worse: less is more. Go lightly with your makeup and know that tomorrow is another day.

THE ASIAN EDGE When an Asian woman wants me to make her eyes look larger, I first make sure she isn't trying to look Caucasian. My makeup philosophy is the same for all women: Don't try to be different, just bring out more of the beauty you already have.

Asian women, typically graced with large, full, expressive faces, often want to make their faces look smaller. I discourage this, stressing my philosophy of enhancing

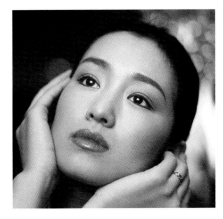

what you've got. If you were born with a round face, a smooth complexion, gorgeous thick dark hair, and almond eyes, count your blessings. These are some of the natural gifts of Asian women, and my advice would be to play them up. In fact, there are some strikingly magnificent Asian faces in film and modeling these days, and that exotic, Eastern image is greatly admired. If you have it, play it up.

Here are some guidelines for Asian makeup:

FOUNDATION: In the past, so many Asian women wore pink-based foundation in an effort to change their skin tone, but pink foundation doesn't work on anyone. A yellow-based foundation is the way to go.

EYEBROWS: Do your brows in a bold way to open the eyes and make them appear larger. It will also add strength to your face, and bring out facial definition.

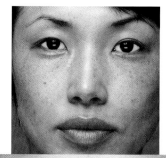

SHADOW: Cover the entire eyelid with shadow to recess the area around the eyes and bringing them out. A medium brown-toned shade blends well with Asian-colored skin tone. If you use two shades, place the darker shade on the bottom part of the lid, blending into a lighter color toward the brow and blend. Lines of shadow demarcation will defeat the sweeping look that opens the eye. Remember: if your shadow is too dark, your eyes will appear diminished in size. Avoid trying to create contour to suggest a larger lid.

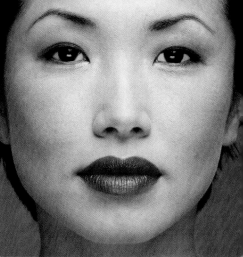

EYELINER: With a pencil, draw a smoky line as close to the lash line as possible. Smudge to open the eye and avoid a harsh look. Make sure your eyeliner can be seen when your eyes are open. Line bottom and top lid, making the bottom lighter and well-blended.

MASCARA: If your eyelashes are sparse, (sometimes the plague of Asian beauty), make it into an advantage by using no mascara at all. Draw attention, instead, to the lash line on the lid, with a smoky eyeliner. If your lashes are full, curl them first, then apply several layers of a black or dark brown mascara. Avoid clumps by combing through after each mascara application.

BLUSH: Apply blush high on the cheeks and sweep it toward the hairline. If your face is full, go lightly on the apple. Play with any color you like. For a more classical look, try the pinker tones. Pale pink looks lovely on pale skin, while rose is nice on darker skin.

LIPS: Experiment with color. Many Asian women are graced with full, well-defined lips and deep tones look sumptuous. Reddish-brown tones will set off your lips beautifully. Extremes can work here, also, as in a pale pink. If you have very full lips, apply lip liner lightly and blend well, or skip it altogether.

- Yellow-based foundation and powder will look the most natural.

- For a full face, dust color lightly on the apple of your cheeks.

- Reddish-brown tones will set off your lips nicely.

HISPANIC AND LATIN "LOOKERS" Latin music is at an all-time height of popularity these days, and the women who represent it are considered to be real "lookers." Think about Jennifer Lopez and Gloria Estefan. Since Latin women have a reputation for being passionate, wild, and exciting, let your makeup reflect it. If that's not you, go for who you are. Don't be stereotyped by expectations.

I have a friend who is a very successful, high-powered businesswoman in the Hispanic community. She always felt she needed to represent the look that people projected onto her, with dark red lips and heavy eyes. I guess she feared that if she strayed from what was expected, she was betraying her culture and her heritage. The problem was that she didn't really feel that red lips and dark makeup reflected the truth about who she was. A modern, fashion-conscious woman, she felt that the darker, heavier look was not really her style, so she had a conflict. She didn't want to appear rebellious to her culture, but at the same time, she wanted to be true to herself.

I advised her to play with her makeup in ways that felt reflective of who she was. She took my advice and she ended up happy with her look.

Guidelines for Latina and Hispanic makeup:

- FOUNDATION: The typical Latina skin has rich orangy-yellow undertones, so find a foundation and a powder that match well with your natural skin tone. Use the same color guidelines if you need to spot your face with concealer. Use bronzing powders to cover blemishes or skin deviations.

- BROWS: Latinas often have very full brows, so making them into thin, little lines would look silly. Wax or tweeze extra hairs that might grow between eyebrows or above and below brow line.

- SHADOW: Look deeply into irises to pick out the best colors. Even with dark eyes, you'll be amazed at the variety of color there when you really look. If your skin has a natural greenish cast, sometimes arising in Hispanic women, use colors that blend well with your foundation. Rose counteracts green, so play with tinted moisturizers. Use darker tones and rich reddish-brown shadows. Go easy with oranges or coral. Think deep, not overly bright. My fine wine color

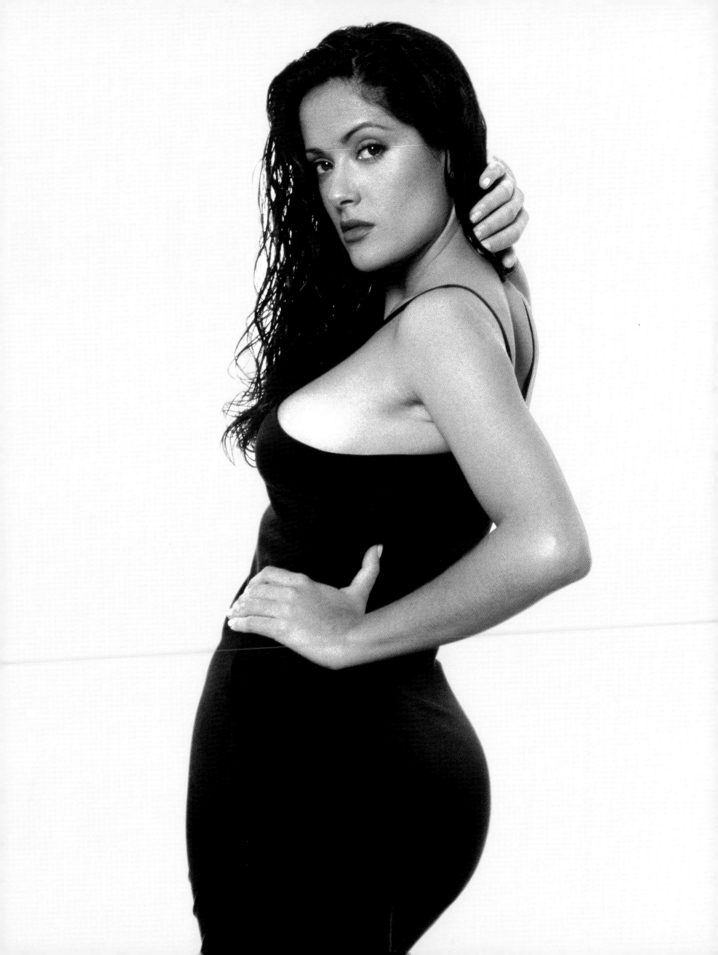

selection would be terrific as would my beautiful naturals collection. Have fun with both.

- EYELINER: Line top and bottom and blend.

- MASCARA: Use black and don't be afraid to layer it on. Comb clumps in between applications, doing bottom lashes as well as the top.

- BLUSH: Sweep the apple with a pop of color to look more alive. Use the same rich tones on the cheeks, moving upward toward the hairline.

- LIPS: Darker reds and wines create a sensuous lip. If your lips are naturally dark, use deep-colored lipsticks with a little bit lighter liner. Again, stay away from oranges and bright shades that pop too much. Line lips subtly or not at all.

HELPFUL HINTS FOR LATINA AND HISPANIC WOMEN:

- Play up your passion.

- Look into irises for shadow color.

- Play with lots of different lip colors.

DARK-SKINNED BEAUTY

I once had a wonderful time making up the Pointer Sisters for an album cover. They were glamorous and fun, and forget stereotypes! They were so open to experimenting with their faces, we all learned a lot that day.

Diana Ross is another example of a beautiful dark-skinned woman who is the epitome of open-minded beauty. In many of her photos, she looks completely different, but always glamorous and true to herself. I'd like to remind dark-skinned women that the shades of your skin can vary greatly from very dark to quite light, so don't get stuck in stereotyping your own skin tone. You can have as much range as a Caucasian woman. Find your own sense of style and express it.

Just for your information, a typical woman of color will be lighter-toned in the cheek area and darker at the chin and brows.

Here are some makeup guidelines for dark-skinned women:

- FOUNDATION: If your skin is even-toned, that's easy. If it isn't, choose a foundation either to bring up the darker tones, or warm the lighter ones. Try a medium foundation color on your entire face. Use a darker one to even out the lighter

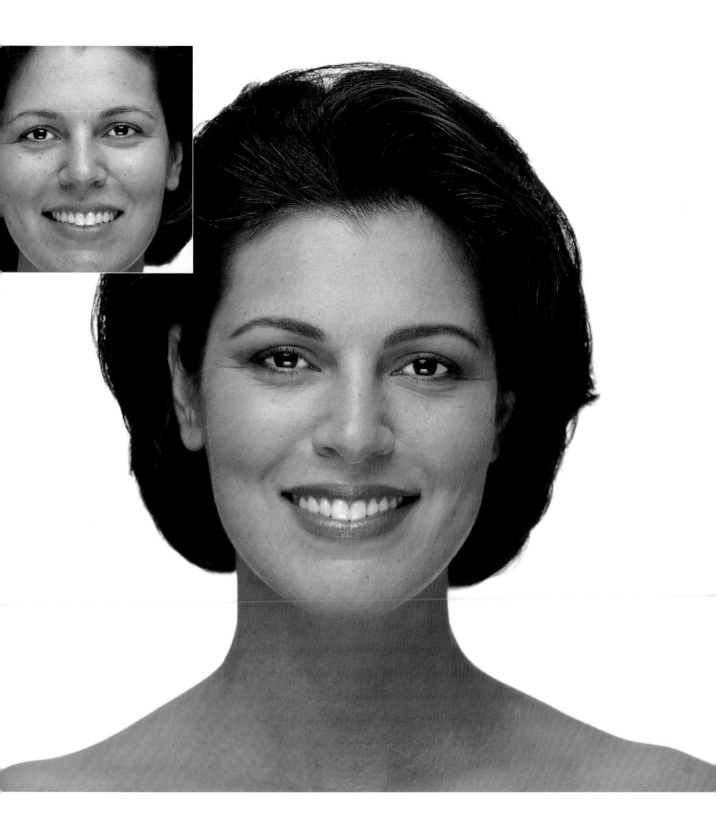

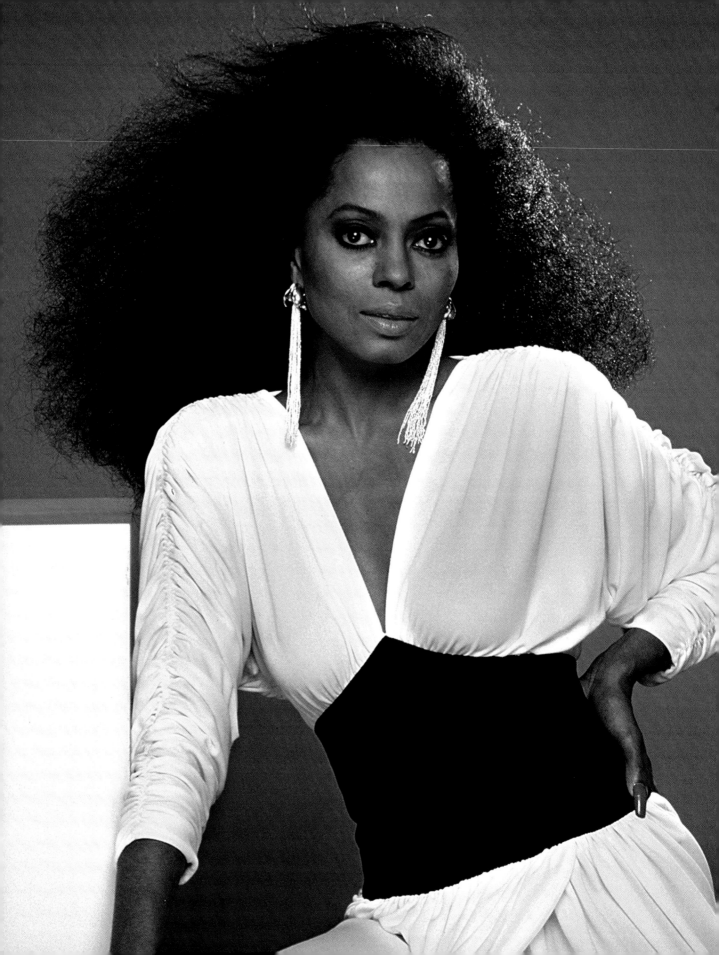

areas. A bronzer can help bring down the lighter skin tones. Use one overall powder to even out the final skin color.

- Brows: Use the natural brow line to frame your face. Use my feathering technique and don't be afraid to accentuate strongly.

- Shadow: Choose a rich color that will blend with your skin. Look into your irises for color choice.

- Eyeliner: A rich dark color will open your eyes and bring out the exotic look. Don't be afraid of nice, strong lines.

- Blush: You may not need blush at all. If you do, pop the apple with a deep reddish tone and use a little darker tone beneath the cheekbones and into the hairline. Stay away from colors that bring out gray, ashy tones on your cheeks.

- Lips: Why do dark-skinned women try to make their lips look smaller while white women are so desperate to pump theirs up? I guess we're used to wanting what we don't have. In order to downplay the size of your lips, eliminate pencil and fill lips in with a subtle color in the soft brown tones. The current trend is a natural, deep brown lip color, with little or no pencil liners.

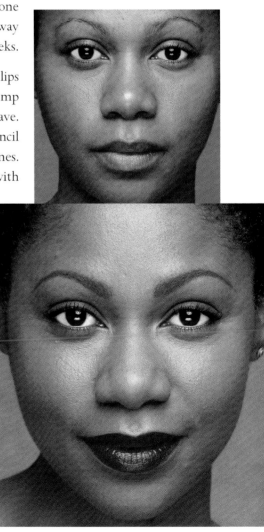

HELPFUL HINTS FOR DARK-SKINNED WOMEN:

- Don't limit your thinking about foundation shades. You have lots of choices.

- If your skin tone is very dark, chances are your lips will be, too. Choose your lip color accordingly.

- Forget about minimizing your lips. Appreciate them and play them to the "fullest."

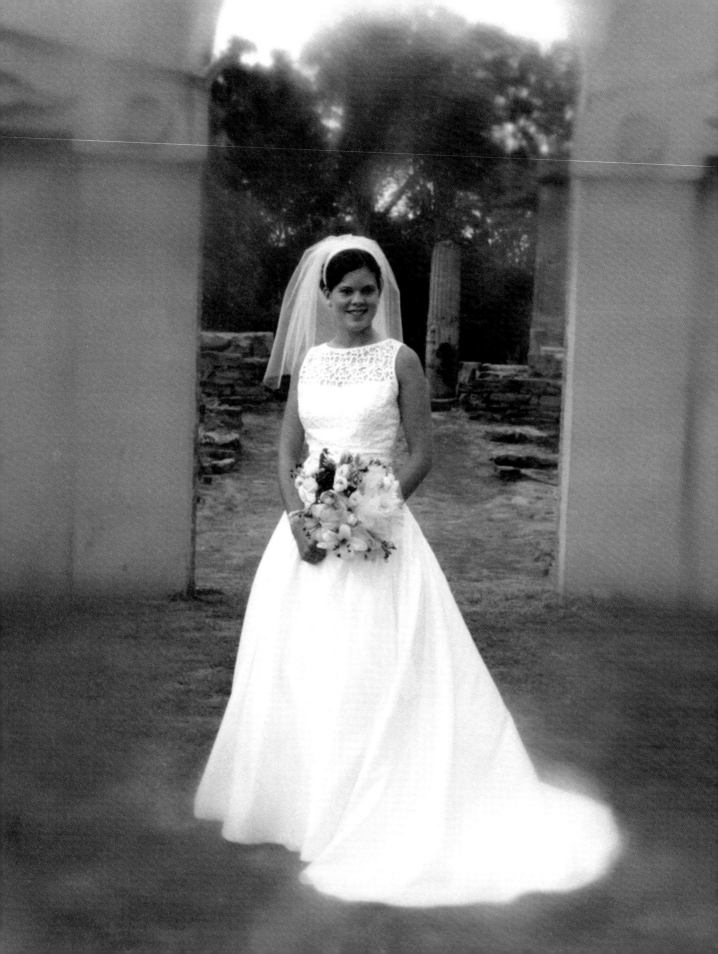

13: KODAK MOMENTS: FROM BLACK TIE TO BABY TIME

THAT KODAK MOMENT You don't need to wear heavy makeup for a picture. In fact, it's better to keep it simple, because the lens does not erase makeup. The same texture that's staring at you through the lens of the camera is exactly what's going to show up in the photograph. Take into consideration whether you'll be indoors or out, and apply makeup according to the light, not the lens.

My initial motivation for creating my foundation was working with actresses and models for film, video, and magazines. When I saw the base shades both through the lens and in the final shots, I wanted something that looked much more natural because electric lights intensify pink. Once again, yellow was where it was.

I learned early on that more was not better, and that it all depended upon application. If you're making up for television, ask the camera operator to roll some tape,

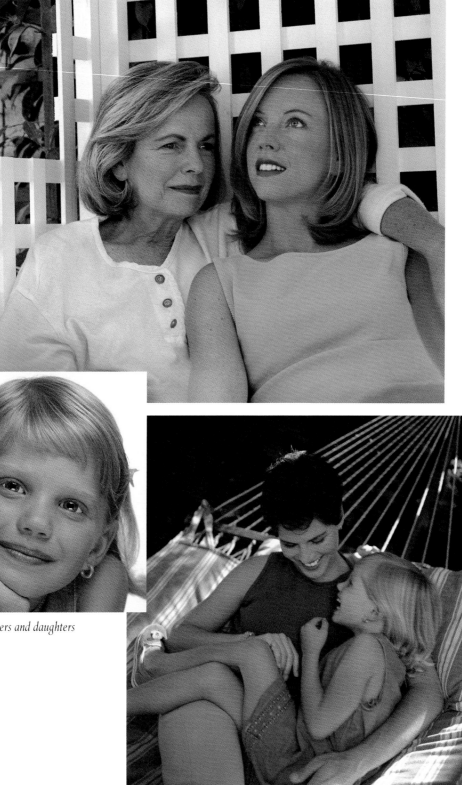

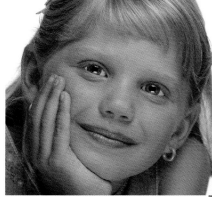

Mothers and daughters

take a look, and decide if that's the way you want to look. For any TV anchors who are reading this book, you don't need to wear so much makeup. It's up to you, not the makeup artist, to decide how you want to present yourself to the world.

If you're going to a family event, a luncheon, or maybe a graduation where someone will be taking pictures, don't change anything. Do your makeup just like you would normally and the photos will come out just fine. For video or film, you can go a little bit heavier because bright light will absorb some of your makeup. Most photography is done in color these days, but for black and white which has more light falling off shadow, you can do a little more contouring.

YOUR PHOTO BAG: Bring a mirror large enough to see your whole face. Include all your essentials as well as eyeliner and lip liner so you can create more perfection for the close-ups. Use your best brushes for a finer touch, and remember your eyelash comb. When a shot gets blown up, lash clumping will be really obvious, and make sure your eyebrows are well groomed for those images frozen in time. Try to avoid the two-minute face. You'll be glad you took the extra time.

THE BIG DATE When you're going out on a first date, remember that makeup sends a message. A softer, subtler face will soften the message. Since first impressions are lasting ones, be yourself. Show off your sense of style and the way you like to carry yourself. If that doesn't cut it, this isn't the guy for you.

Taking some time for your makeup will make you less apprehensive. Approach it logically, considering where you're going and the time of day. Heavy makeup and dark colors are obviously off track for the beach or taking a hike out in nature. Remember that over-compensating creates a look that isn't really you. Have fun with your face, but remember to present the most beautiful and natural you. Your date is interested in you, not your makeup, so don't hide your face. You want to show up looking great and feeling great, so you can forget about your makeup and just have a good time. Remember, you'll be meeting *him* for the first time, too, and you want to be able to see who you're with instead of worrying about looking all right.

For one of my infomercials, I interviewed a number of sexy, hot guys about what they liked and didn't like about makeup. The vote was almost unanimous that heavy makeup was a turn-off. This is good to remember for women in their forties, fifties, and even sixties who are still dating. Caking on the makeup to hide lines is not the way to go. If he doesn't appreciate your hard-earned character, it's time to move on.

YOUR DATE BAG: Take some makeup with you for touch-ups: foundation, blush, mascara, and lipstick. Bring some tissues in case you go dancing and need to pat dry your face or clean your eyes.

MARRIAGE MAGIC On your wedding day, you are the star. Everyone's going to be looking at you, so you want to feel really good about that. Sometimes that's easier said than done. I remember at my wedding, when I began my walk down the aisle, and everyone stood up. I was shocked. I wasn't used to being the center of attention and thought, "Gee, everyone is staring at me. I hope I look pretty."

Feeling confident about your makeup is one way to feel more relaxed during this intense time. The best advice I can offer brides is that your groom proposed to YOU, and you are the one he wants to marry. If he sees a stranger standing next to him, he'll probably feel uncomfortable.

More important, you need to feel comfortable. Getting married is one of the most memorable events of your life. You'll be reminded about it over and over, often in a video, and certainly in photographs. Since you want to put the most beautiful "you" on display, your wedding is not the time to try out a brand new look. It's time to do a makeup that's more refined and perfected, but not necessarily different or heavier. Think pretty, classic, and up close. If you've hired a professional makeup artist for the event, try her out at least a week beforehand. If you like her work, you're all set. If you don't, you'll still have time to look further. Why would you run the risk of hating the way your face looks ten minutes before you're scheduled to walk down the aisle?

Take plenty of time to prepare for your wedding. Obvious, right? You'd be surprised how many women fly into the ceremony in a panic, flustered and unsure about how they look. Take a long bath with sweet smelling subtle fragrances, (think flowers, not flower shops so you don't bowl over your groom), and have adequate time and the right people around. Place dots of fragrance behind the ears, on wrists, and behind the knees. You can spray a fine mist of fragrance into the air and walk through it to provide a head to toe scent.

The focus for wedding makeup is your eyes. It's all about connection—looking into your groom's eyes. A wedding ceremony is extremely intimate, and you want your eyes to look as beautiful as possible, never overdone. Since many weddings take place in the daytime, you probably don't want your makeup to be overly dramatic. Don't focus on the party afterward—one thing at a time. Your ultimate goal is to feel pretty and comfortable at the moment. Then you can put your attention on the experience and on your groom, instead of worrying if your eyes look all right.

This is not the time to bring your foundation and powder all the way down your neckline. A layer of makeup around the neck edge of your dress will not be an added attraction. Use powder to make sure there's no shine, because it really shows up in pictures.

Choose the softer shadow colors, preferably in earth tones. Keep it light and lovely, avoiding fuchsias and heavy iridescents, but a sprinkle of shimmer around the eyes can be beautiful. As a general rule, use colors that make you feel safe and comfortable as opposed to wild and provocative. Think about your surroundings when you choose your colors, such as walls and floral arrangements. If you wear white as many brides do, your cheeks may need some extra color to avoid looking washed out.

Your face may be naturally flushed, so go easy with your blush. I'd stay away from high contrast and use a color that matches your clothing as well as your surroundings and remember to blend it really well. A 10 AM outdoor wedding will take place in different light than one at 4 PM, so plan your makeup accordingly. Whichever time and setting you choose, this is clearly the time for waterproof mascara. Nobody gets through a wedding, particularly her own, without at least one good cry, and some women cry all the way through it. One good layer of waterproof mascara will be sufficient with a thorough comb-through afterward to remove clumps.

These days, women are comfortable enough to walk down the aisle not only in traditional wedding gowns, but also in nontraditional colors and styles of clothing. This is partly because women are marrying at all ages and not necessarily for the first time. Whether you're wearing white, ivory, black, or any shade in between, make sure your makeup, in this case, your eye shadow, complements your clothing. For darker bridal wear, you can handle a slightly heavier makeup application, than when wearing pristine white. If you want to get married in something besides the traditional white gown, feel free to do it. The important thing is that on this special day of your life, your clothing and your makeup should reflect the beautiful woman that you truly are.

I suggest a natural lip stain, one that won't come off during that important kiss. Keep away from lip gloss. Try a sheer color, this is not the time for big, bold, red, heavily outlined lips. Not only will it look unnatural, it could stain your wedding gown. Pinks and peaches work very well, (if you're wearing white), or any other color that blends well with what you're wearing and with the rest of your makeup.

For the reception or party afterward, you can intensify and darken your lips, especially if you're going to be changing clothes. This is when you can have a little bit more fun with colors.

Keep in mind that your makeup doesn't have to last for eight hours. Touch-ups are not only allowed for brides, they're expected, a great excuse to take a break in the middle of a busy time that's basically focused on you.

YOUR BRIDAL BAG: Let your maid of honor carry a bridal bag that contains what you'll need for touch-ups. Bring some foundation with a sponge and some pressed powder with a puff. (Avoid carrying loose powder that can open in your purse.) Include blush, a brown eye pencil, and waterproof mascara. Have a light, sheer lipstick for the early part of the day, long-lasting if possible, and a darker shade with some iridescence if you like, as the day progresses. (Some iridescence in the center of your lips highlights and fills them out.) If you have a favorite scent, include that with a good luck charm or a crystal. It can't hurt!

PREGNANCY Being pregnant can be an exquisite time in your life, but it can also be extremely challenging. Some women feel fabulous the whole time, which makes me so envious. Although my three pregnancies were wonderful in their own special ways, I had a lot of morning sickness. Needless to say, looking good was the last thing I thought about when I was crouched over the toilet. Makeup was optional during this time, a day-to-day decision based upon how I felt.

No matter how it unfolds, being pregnant carries with it such a sense of awe and wonder. Everything is changing, especially your hormones which can drive your moods, so it's important to be kind to yourself. Allow yourself to experience the natural changes that will be sweeping through you without any extra demands. If you don't feel like wearing makeup, don't. If you feel particularly well one day and wearing makeup seems like fun, have a good time. It may make you feel better during your pregnancy, because odd things sometimes happen to your skin.

When I was pregnant, especially the last time, I noticed an unevenness in my skin tone. I compensated by mixing my foundation a little bit darker than usual. I found out later that my problem was called "melasma," or what's known as "the mask of pregnancy." A hormonal condition, this often happens to women with dark hair and dark eyes, so my foundation was a great help until it evened back out.

Some women get dry skin during this time, while others become uncharacteristically oily and break out. Some women have the most fabulous peaches-and-cream complexion, and others look a little green. Makeup can brighten you up and make you feel better during this period of inconsistency. It can also be reassuring if you feel heavy or sexually unattractive. In this culture, we all want to think we're desirable. When our stomachs expand, our skin gets strange, and our faces plump out, we women need reminders that we still look beautiful. I gained forty pounds with each pregnancy, and it really showed in my face. If this happens to you, don't panic. Makeup can help. Don't worry, I lost the weight each time, so I know you can.

Try a little facial contouring if you need it, but don't overdo it. There's a tendency to want to sculpt back the cheekbones that seem to have disappeared, but it'll only make things worse. Just cover inconsistencies and brighten up your face. A natural glow seems to show up in a pregnant woman's face, especially toward the end, and you need to celebrate it. Real life will return soon enough with little time for anything, so enjoy this phase and revel in it. By the way, if you don't have that "natural glow, " create it with blush.

BABY TIME Once you have the baby, forget about makeup for the first week or two. You'll be lucky if you find time to take a shower or run a comb through your hair. After the first couple of weeks, while you're in a sleep-deprived state and falling in love with the newest member of the family, you'll bless the two-minute face—if you can find two minutes.

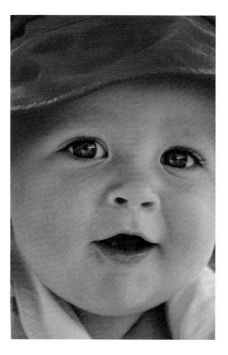

You'll be glad you did your homework, because there is virtually no time to experiment. You'll be rushing to throw on your face while the baby naps, and believe me, he or she will do it on his or her own time, not yours. They just don't understand that you need an extra moment to use your lip liner. The days of standing in the bathroom for thirty minutes are over. Each second you have to do something for yourself really counts, so go back to Chapter Ten and review the Two-Minute Face.

For your Baby Bag, throw a few things of your own into the diaper bag. Include whatever will give you a lift and an instant result so you can feel a little bit more pulled together. I suggest a lipstick and a little bit of blush. Anything more will probably go unused and just take up space.

BLACK-TIE BLOWOUT Pull out the fun drawer! It's time to rock! Since your clothes will be more dramatic and it will most likely be evening light, take license to have a ball with your makeup. Think glamour and elegance! I didn't say to overdo it, though. For black-tie events, since your clothes often make a powerful statement, you don't want your makeup distracting from them. Create a balance. If you're planning a dramatic face, focus on one particular feature to which you want to draw attention. For example, if you want to create a sensuous, exciting mouth, make your eyes strong but downplay them in relationship to your lips. Keep in mind that the cooler the tones, the stronger the contrast, which definitely suggests a dramatic look.

Avoid trying to create a porcelain skin or a dark tan with your foundation. Stick to what matches your skin tone and play up your features. I pull out my liquid eyeliner at these times to create a little more depth around my eyes, which adds a sense of drama. You can intensify your eyebrows a little bit more than usual, and use an extra layer or two of mascara. Since most black-tie events are in artificial light, shimmer around the eyes will look great. It's time to go upscale, and what's more exciting than red, shiny lips? Keep in mind that one feature accentuated, with the rest supporting the look, will be eye-stopping.

Don't put pressure on yourself. There's a lot more flexibility with black tie these days than there used to be. Remember that dramatic makeup doesn't necessarily mean heavy makeup. If your gown is elegant and intricate, try a simple makeup with your hair pulled back away from your face. Black-tie, at its best, is all about classic, timeless beauty. Princess Diana was famous for this; she often let her gown make the statement, supported by high heels, slicked-back hair, and a soft and dramatic makeup.

A word of caution: A hairdresser once asked me if she could try something on me for a black-tie event, a version of pinning my hair on top of my head. I was wary, but I decided to let her go for it. I ended up with a very dated look, my hair piled high on my head with crazy curls sticking out all over the place. I left the salon thinking I looked like my mother, thirty years ago, but I decided to ignore it, mainly because I had no time to change it. The worst part of the evening was when my husband walked past me at the event where I was meeting him. And then there was the expression on his face when he realized it was me. I was stuck with that look, and it turned out to be a very uncomfortable evening.

The moral of the story is: Try out a new look beforehand, with plenty of time to change it if you don't like it.

YOUR BLACK-TIE BAG: This is the time for a little jeweled compact with your favorite powder shade. Include in your bag small pots of foundation, powder, blush, mascara, lipstick, and don't forget lip pencil so your lipstick lasts and doesn't bleed into fine lines. Coco Chanel said that fragrance was one of the most important parts of creating a sophisticated, elegant look, and I agree. I have some nighttime fragrances in my line that I take with me to black-tie events. Then, I can put a little on my wrists, behind the ears, and behind my knees when I do my touch-ups.

- There's plenty of time for touch-ups after a wedding ceremony and before photographs, so you don't have to do an eight-hour makeup.

- A little iridescence in the center of your lips highlights and fills out your lips.

- Use foundation to cover skin inconsistencies during pregnancy.

- After the baby is born, go back to Chapter Ten and review the Two-Minute Face.

- Create a makeup that makes you feel comfortable on a first date. Avoid caking or covering with heavy foundation.

- Shimmer is terrific for black-tie events. Think classic, elegant, and sophisticated.

BEAUTY MARK

1:

For your wedding, make up your face to look like you. Your husband
doesn't want to marry somebody else.

BEAUTY MARK

2:

Makeup sends a message for that first date. Be yourself.

BEAUTY MARK

3:

One feature accentuated, with the rest supporting the look,
will be eye-stopping.

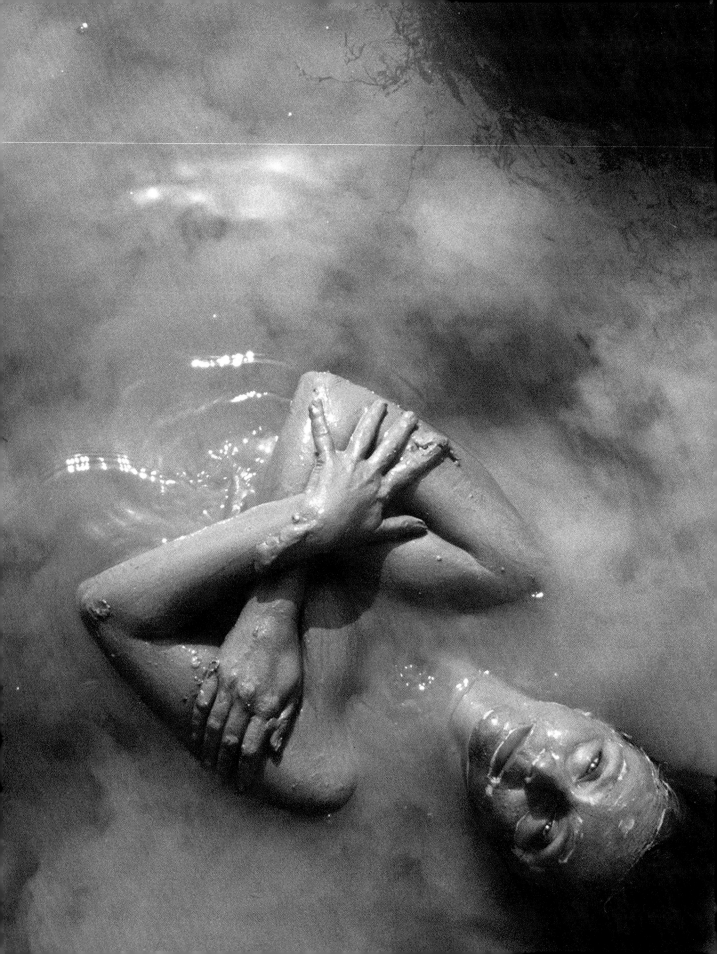

14: SKIN CARE: LOTIONS & POTIONS

SKIN BASICS Beauty is reflected from the inside out. The quality of your skin will reflect the health of your organs. The skin, which is basic to your bodily functions, helps you breathe, sense, ventilate, excrete, and defend the system against diseases. A healthy skin, even if it isn't flawless, will not only look better, it also will help regulate your body temperature, store nutrients, and protect you against the elements. It is your skin that reflects your state of beauty, making it the most multifunctional organ you have. Yes, it's an organ, just like your liver, heart, or kidneys. Since your skin sheds and regenerates monthly, if you make a concerted effort, you can see a tremendous difference in as little as thirty days.

If you weren't born with great skin, don't despair. Genetics play a large part here, but having imperfect skin doesn't mean you can't dramatically improve your skin's appearance by caring for it well. To some extent, we all have sensitivities to certain plants and chemicals, so it's your individual job to figure out how sensitive your skin is, what type you have, and how best to care for it.

CLEANSING AND YOUR SKIN TYPE Take a moment in the morning when you are free of makeup before your shower or bath, to discover your particular skin type. This will make all the difference in determining your most optimum cleansing and maintenance routine. Lightly clean your face with a mild cleanser, pat dry, and then press a tissue lightly on the facial skin around your nose, forehead, cheeks, and chin. Now study the skin on your face:

- NORMAL SKIN HAS NO OVERLY SHINY AREAS. It basically feels good most of the time and will leave little or no residue on the tissue. Use a water-soluble cleanser or a cleansing milk.

- OILY OR ACNE-PRONE SKIN IS SHINY ALL OVER. The tissue will have residue from all the areas you test. Use a gel or lotion cleanser containing salicylic acid which clears out bacteria build-up that causes breakouts.

- DRY SKIN LOOKS TIGHT AND FEELS FLAKY. It will leave no residue deposits on the tissue. Use a gentle cleansing milk or water-soluble cleanser that leaves a light emollient on the skin's surface to soothe dryness.

- COMBINATION SKIN LEAVES OIL ON THE TISSUE FROM YOUR FOREHEAD, NOSE, AND CHIN (THAT'S CALLED THE T-ZONE). Your cheek area, which is dryer on almost everyone, will deposit no residue at all. Use a foaming cleanser or a cleansing lotion with salicylic acid, focusing on the T-zone.

Now that you know your skin type, which may change slightly with your menstrual cycle and hormonal fluctuations, you can determine the right cleansing routine. Note the following and make the appropriate adjustments:

- In summer, your skin is generally drier on the surface, oilier underneath.

- In winter, your skin is often dry all the way through.

- Around the holidays, your skin tends to be oilier.

- If you travel on planes a great deal or for an extended flight, the recycled air will dry out your skin.

I designed my cleansing program to be effective and time-saving. Before I share it with you, let me break down in more detail the types of cleansers that are currently available in the marketplace.

With the advantage of modern technology, many of today's cleansing products are designed not only to remove surface dirt, but also to protect the face and add radi-

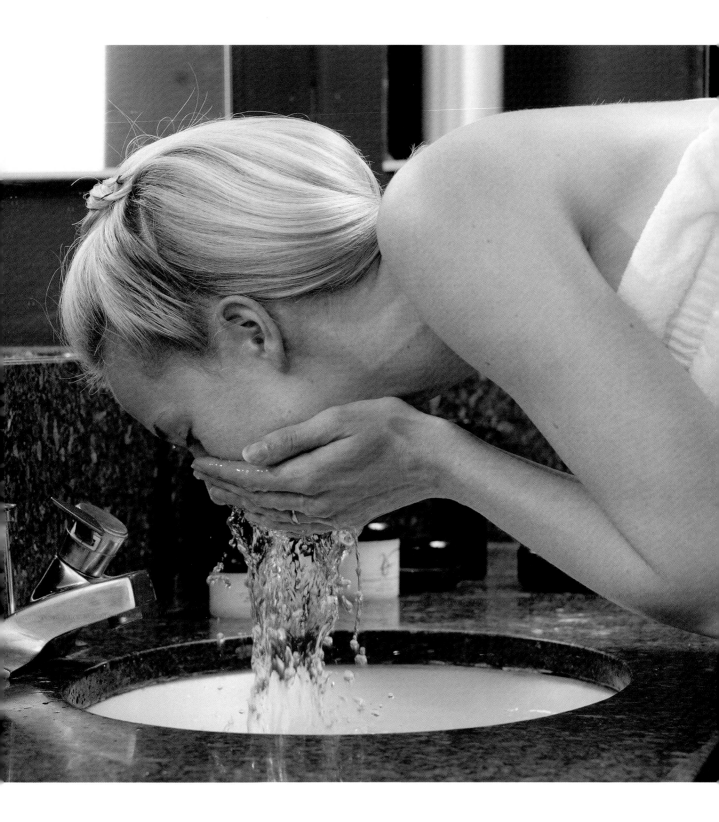

ance with vitamins, sunscreens, antioxidants, exfoliants, and emollients. Here's a list of the various types and what kind of skin to which they are best suited:

- WATER-SOLUBLE CLEANSERS: All purpose, good for general cleansing with all skin types. This is my favorite. The formula I sell in my line. It's nonirritating, cleans the skin well, and leaves it feeling soft and smooth.

- GEL CLEANSERS: Oil-free and less alkaline than soap. Recommended for oily and combination skin.

- LOTION CLEANSERS: Good for dry and sensitive skin, since they contain mild moisturizers that leave a light film to soothe the face.

- FOAMING CLEANSERS: Perfect for combination skin as this type is gentle enough for normal skin and strong enough for an oily T-zone.

- CLEANSING MILKS: Available in three forms with ingredients designed for all types of skin.

- OIL-FREE CLEANSING LOTIONS: Often contain glycolic acid for exfoliation. They work well for combination skin that isn't too sensitive.

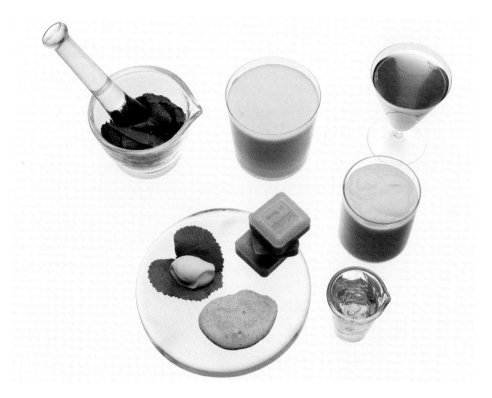

A few guidelines for skin cleansing:

- Cleanse and moisturize your face twice a day, morning and evening.

- Remove all makeup each night with a makeup remover, a cleanser, or a two-in-one.

- To get the first layer of cleanser off your face, a soft washcloth or cotton pad dipped in warm water will do the trick. Then splash with warm water several times to get it really clean.

A word about pores: Oily skin can draw attention to oversized pores. Keep your skin clean and free from extra oil, and consult a dermatologist for topical agents or prescribed medications to reduce pore appearance.

EXFOLIATING THE OUTER LAYERS

The purpose of an exfoliant is to slough off old, excess skin cells from the epidermal surface. When used properly, the results will be a smoother, more even skin, due to exposed new cells that have been hiding underneath. When you exfoliate as needed, your pores can better absorb moisturizers and your makeup will cover more evenly. Just remember: ALWAYS BE GENTLE WITH EXFOLIANTS.

Let me remind you that if you're looking for miracle de-aging products, you'll probably go broke and crazy before you ever find what you're looking for. I'm not saying that there aren't products that can help. Many women can tolerate ingredients like glycolic acid and Retin-A, which create cellular skin turnover, exfoliating the top layers, and eventually give you a healthier, newer-looking skin. For those who can use them, after a period of redness, a wonderful glow can arise from underneath. Many women love this approach, so I put some of these ingredients in my line, but, as with all skin products, test them on a small area of your skin for several days to see how you react. Some people, myself included, find them too irritating, even in the most minute amounts.

There are a large number of ways to achieve skin exfoliation from gently using a washcloth to strong serums that contain alpha-hydroxy acid (AHAs). Choose your exfoliation method according to your skin sensitivity, how often you wish to exfoliate, if you want to clear up acne, if you wish to reduce the appearance of fine lines, or if you want to clean up your skin's texture or coloration. Here is what's available today:

- FACIAL SCRUBS: In gel and cleanser forms, these contain fine particles that loosen the dead skin cells. Rub them GENTLY on the skin, rinse them off, and the old cells will be gone.

- Buffing Creams: Stronger than a facial scrub. Leave on for five to ten minutes and slough off GENTLY in a circular motion.

- Exfoliating Masks: Massage these GENTLY into the skin for a few seconds, and rinse off. This will work well for both normal and sensitive skin.

- AHAs or Fruit Acids: Found in gel, lotion, and facial mask formulas, these are a brand new breed of exfoliant. Good for oily skin because you can avoid scrubbing which stimulates acne flare-ups.

- Tretinoin: Available by prescription only, this is a vitamin-derived solution (the brand name is Retin-A) that helps shed dead skin cells. This very drying chemical dissolves the top layer of skin. Please use only under the supervision of a dermatologist, be sure to use a good moisturizer, and KEEP OUT OF THE SUN.

- Silk Mitts or Synthetic Loofahs: Manual exfoliants that help shed dead skin cells. The mitt is less abrasive, so use GENTLY on face, especially for dry skin. Loofahs are good for the entire body.

MOISTURIZERS: WHICH ONE AND WHEN

Everyone doesn't always need to use a moisturizer all over the face. If your skin is naturally oily, a moisturizer could clog the pores. You see, a moisturizer doesn't really soak into the skin, itself. Rather, it creates a barrier between the air and your skin, keeping your natural moisture from evaporating. When water is trapped in your skin, it plumps out and takes on a lovely, smooth appearance.

> *I'm a real fan of moisturizer. I always keep some with me, for those little dry spots that can come up during the day.*
> *—Lisa Hartman*

Using moisturizers is a good way to relieve itchiness and irritation, since they contain ingredients that temporarily repair damaged skin. You can spot moisturizer, like foundation, on such dry areas as the cheeks. As we get older, though, most of us need to cover the entire face.

Here's the list:

- Oil-Containing Moisturizers: These use a large array of oils including, vegetable, mineral, and animal-type.

- Oil-Free Moisturizers: These come in lightweight lotions and gels. They contain mucopolysaccharides and hyluronic acid, nonabsorbable chemicals which form a water-binding film on the surface of the skin.

- Glycerin: A humectant that attracts water and hydrates chapped skin.

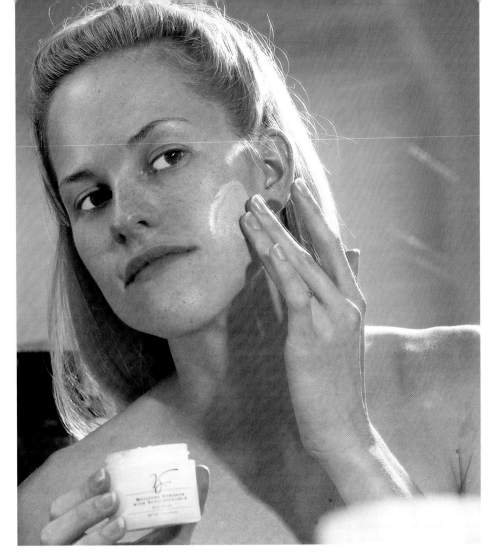

If your skin is normal, use a light, water-based formula. For oily skin, use an oil-free formula. Combination skins respond best to lightweight, water-based formulas, while dry skin responds to a moisturizer with heavier emollients.

If the highly sensitive area beneath your eyes tends to be dry, you may want to use an eye cream. It works wonders on that delicate skin, and can be used daily. Try a gel form when you need to reduce puffiness.

PLANNING YOUR PERSONAL SKIN-CARE ROUTINE
Time often feels like the enemy, doesn't it? I rarely find more than a few minutes in the morning or the evening, so I need a fast and effective skin-care routine that leaves my skin feeling and looking clean. Since caring for the skin is the first and most important step in an effective beauty regimen, let me tell you what I do.

My basic skin-care routine:

STEP 1: In the morning, I wash my face with my gentle cleanser, which dissolves excess oily build-up from overnight and kills any accumulating bacteria.

STEP 2: (optional) I use a scrub when needed. I always make sure the granules are extremely fine and non-abrasive.

STEP 3: Then I use my toner which contains collagen, Elastin, and Aloe Vera to stimulate the skin, refine the pores, and get rid of minute traces of cleanser.

STEP 4: Finally, I use my light moisturizer which contains sunscreen. If I'm going to be caught in the sun, I always make sure to wear a wide-brimmed hat and I put sunscreen on the vulnerable parts of my body. I plan events like walks and gardening when the rays are not directly overhead.

In the evening, I follow almost the same cleansing routine as I do in the morning. The main difference is that I've had makeup on all day, so removing it completely with something that treats my skin nicely, is my first concern. That's why I created my cleanser to be dual-action—a makeup remover and a soothing facial cleanser in one. It feels like I'm using water, it completely removes my makeup, and leaves next to no residue.

My experience is that my skin secretes natural oils while I sleep, so I use a light touch with my moisturizer, both morning and evening. Just make sure you remove your makeup completely every night, which allows your skin to breathe during sleep. Then you'll wake up with a clean, radiant face (and your eyelashes won't break off). By the way, in the evening, for the last step, I apply my night cream sparingly, which obviously contains no sunscreen. Some skin care specialists suggest a heavier moisturizer at night. If that feels good to you, go ahead. For me, I always like a lighter cream.

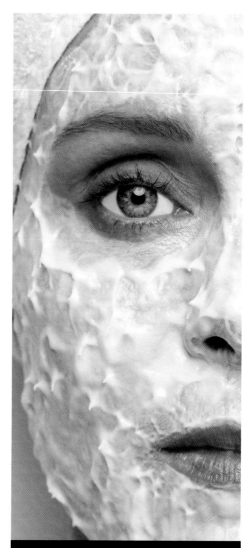

I call Victoria's makeup remover "magic water." I've used it for years, because makeup is such a big part of my life.

— Vanna White

When needed and when time permits, I either see a facialist or I apply my facial masque which tightens and refines the pores, ridding the skin surface of any accumulated dead cells. Mine is in gel form, but there are a variety of masks on the market, including oatmeal, mud, clay, aloe vera, cucumber, and so many more. Play with them and choose one that gives you the desired results.

Applying a mask as needed or desired is a great excuse to relax because you can't answer the phone or the door with a green or a blue mask drying on your face (at least, I don't). As far as actual skin benefits, masks reduce the size of the pores, they create a cell tightening which makes you look fresh and young, and they just plain feel good. I try to do them as often as possible, because I really notice the difference during particularly busy weeks when I find no time for extra pampering.

TANNING YOUR HIDE In the 1920s, when Coco Chanel declared that a tan was chic and a sign of affluence, she had no idea she was starting one of the most destructive fashion trends in history. There's very little difference between baking your oiled face in the sun, and the way a tanner dries out animal hides for clothing or furniture. If you choose a soft, lovely facial skin over a leathery one that feels like cowhide, stay out of the sun—and out of tanning salons. They all claim to be safe, but since there are no regulations in this country, most of them have proven to be quite harmful, long-term. Let's just be grateful that having a tanned face is no longer "in."

If the word "sunscreen" makes you want to run, take heart. Remember when they used to irritate your skin and your eyes? They've come a long way in the past few years, with lighter, effective formulas that are far less irritating, nongreasy, and long-lasting. Keep in mind that sun damage happens when you least expect it. Just because you wear sunscreen at the beach doesn't mean you're "covered." What about in the car on the way there, when the sun comes streaming in the windows? Or when the sun is hiding behind the clouds, but the damaging UVA light that causes melanin spotting, photo-aging, and cancer still makes it through?

IMPORTANT GUIDELINES FOR SUNSCREEN:

- SPF numbers can be misleading. In tests, an SPF 15 absorbed 93% of the sun's damaging rays, while an SPF 30 absorbed 97%. The FDA suggests that with anything over 30, the extra protection is negligible.

- Skin on the face and the body require different types of sunscreens.

- For breakout-prone skin, use sunscreen in oil-free gels or spray formulas. For dry skin, creamier formulas will work out fine. If your skin is still too sensitive for sunscreen, there are now formulas for babies that you'll most likely be able to tolerate.

- Check your makeup. Some of today's formulas contain sunscreen, but higher SPF numbers combined with foundation can create irritation.

- Apply sunscreen liberally thirty minutes before sun exposure to give your skin time to absorb it.

- Reapply after swimming, sweating, or toweling off.

- Don't forget that your lips need sunscreen, too. Some lipsticks contain SPF 25, and so do many lip balms.

- The skin around your eyes needs a formula that was created specifically for its delicacy and proximity to eyes. No fragrances or other common irritants allowed in this area.

- Choose sunglasses with UVA and UVB ray protection for your eyes.

Keep in mind that if you're using Retin-A, or if you had a facial chemical peel, plastic surgery, or you're taking medications that create skin sensitivity, you must use sunscreen without fail any time you go outdoors or sit by windows. Let's keep that skin feeling, looking, and acting like skin!

"MIRACLE" CLAIMS Regarding products that make impossible claims: No skin care item can actually work miracles. If you want to see a miracle and you still smoke cigarettes, quit smoking. In a very short period of time, watch feathery lines in your skin diminish! Not only does your skin react to nicotine by eventually taking on a yellowish cast, but pursing of your lips to inhale the smoke also creates permanent lines around your lips.

Certain products can create the illusion of diminishing fine lines, but nothing removes wrinkles permanently. Just keep your skin clean, avoid sun damage, which can be terrifically aging, and love the way you look. And you might reread the anecdote about Bette Davis's attitude toward wrinkles in Chapter one.

If you can afford it, see a facialist once a month. This is not only great for your skin, it's also very relaxing for your mind and your spirit. If you can't manage the expense, try doing it once or twice a year and be extra diligent about your cleansing routines.

HELPFUL HINTS:

- There are no anti-aging miracle products. Don't be fooled by false claims and keep your money in your purse.

- Follow a short skin-care routine, morning and evening, that leaves your skin feeling clean and fresh, ready for makeup or a good night's sleep.

- Completely remove all makeup at night. Leaving your mascara on while you sleep will weaken eyelashes, causing them to break off.

- A gentle, regular habit of skin exfoliation, that is, sloughing off old, dead skin cells, will make the skin smoother as it exposes the hidden newer cells.

- An eye gel will help reduce puffiness on that delicate under-eye area.

- Sunscreen is vital to prevent damage and skin cancer. Use different formulas for your face and your body.

BEAUTY MARK
1:
If you like using soap, make sure your brand isn't drying. Remember: what worked at sixteen, doesn't necessarily work at forty.

BEAUTY MARK
2:
Use facial scrubs sparingly and only as needed. Large granules break skin capillaries and so does vigorous scrubbing.

BEAUTY MARK
3:
I find that a heavy sunscreen can cause breakouts, so I lightly cover my skin with my foundation which has a built-in sunscreen that doesn't create irritation.

SKIN CARE: LOTIONS & POTIONS

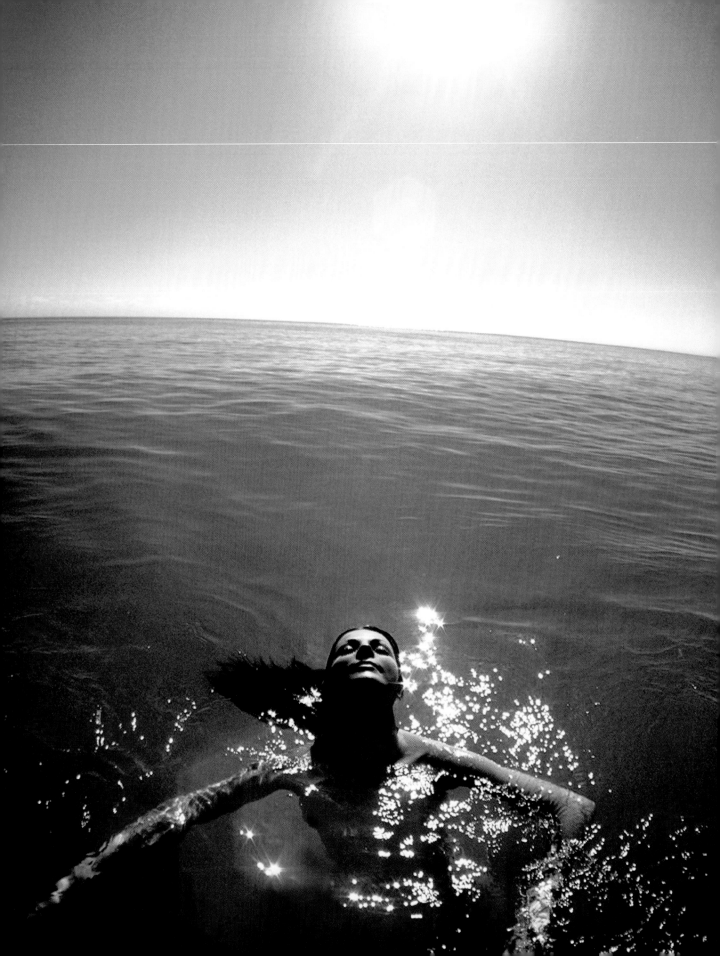

15: MOVING, EATING, & RELAXING

BLENDING BEAUTY WITH GOOD HEALTH

FITNESS, NUTRITION, AND RELAXATION are inextricably woven together. The combination of a good exercise program, a healthy diet, and some time set aside to close your eyes and just "be," will most assuredly make you look better physically and feel better emotionally. We all know by now that plenty of sleep, healthy grooming routines, lots of water, and fresh nutritious foods will give our skin that healthy glow by improving its texture, moisture levels, and sensitivity. The question is, did you know that the same elements will also greatly affect your mental attitude?

There are so many ways to get your body and mind in shape these days, excuses simply don't hold water. You either care enough about yourself to make the effort or you don't. If you're someone who really wants to get it together but you can't seem to take the first step, I can relate. I always hated exercise programs that were rigid—you know, an hour of lifting weights two to three times a week, a boring, exhausting kind of aerobics four or five times a week, and food deprivation, to boot. When I actually managed to show up for these things, I spent the time watching the clock. When I didn't make it, I felt guilty. Is this familiar? How about the expensive piece of equipment you ordered at New Year's on the heels of your resolutions, that's gathering dust or taking up space in your home?

We've all made resolutions that we didn't keep, so let's lighten up and just think about being healthy and feeling and looking good. To achieve this, moderation in exercise and food is a smart goal. As I get older, I'm aware of feeling tired and of the lack of glow on my skin when I don't get to the gym, when I eat junk food, when I lose sleep, or when I'm overly stressed about business or family. I've also noticed a radiance in my face and a dramatic rise in my energy when I exercise regularly, eat nutritiously, sleep well, and keep my stress levels down. The older we get, the less we can kid ourselves that it doesn't matter. It really does.

STRETCHING AND STAYING CENTERED Since Ali MacGraw worked
with me on my first infomercial, I've been inspired with how centered she seems to be. Even when the craziness of her life was at its peak, I saw how her Yoga practice kept her on track. Ali was way ahead of her time by using the meditative aspects of Yoga to quiet her mind. I was initially intimidated by her dedication to her practice. I kept myself away from it by saying things like, "I'm not as flexible as she is," or "I don't have her body." When I stopped the excuses and starting going to Yoga classes, I realized that just because I can't bend over backward and twist myself into a pretzel, doesn't mean I can't quiet my mind and feel better.

Remember: flexibility equals youthful feelings. Nothing makes you feel old faster than when your joints hurt and your walk reflects a hunched-over slow-moving gait. Regular stretching keeps the spine straight, helps prevent muscles from appearing bulky, and creates a sleeker, more elegant look to your body. It also strengthens your muscles, it feels great, and you can even do it in bed! As you get older, stretching will also support your body in such a way to prevent you from falling down and breaking bones. With all these benefits and next to no detriments, what have you got to lose?

For overall beauty, I take fanatically good care of my skin, both with skin care and with diet, Yoga, stress-relief, etc.

— *Ali MacGraw*

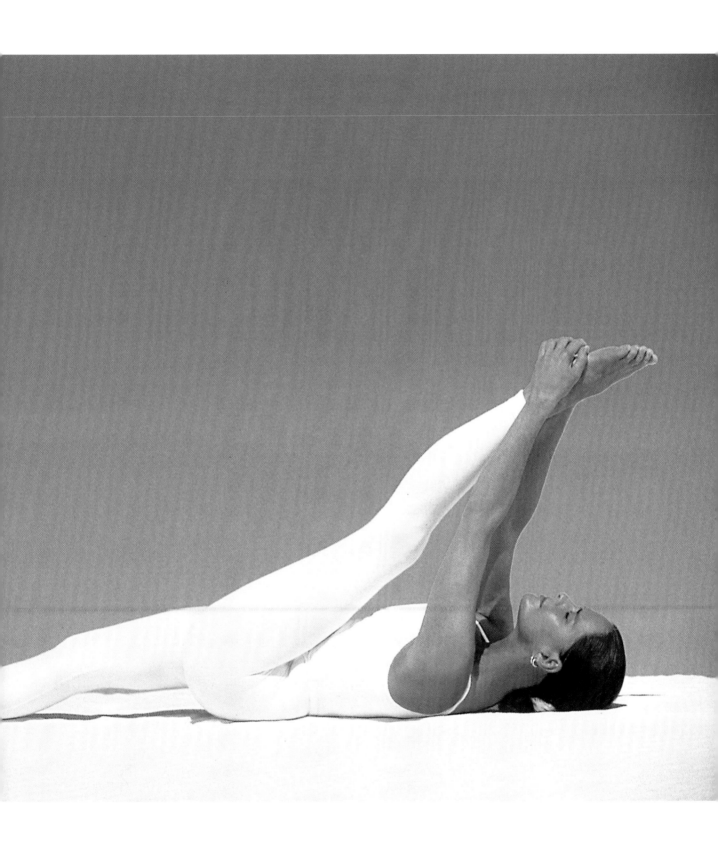

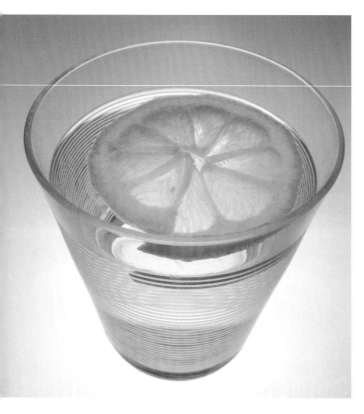

WATER, GOOD FOOD, AND MORE WATER

If you're like me, you know you're supposed to drink water, but you just don't always get around to it. Nutritionists recommend 6 to 8 glasses of water a day. If you can get in the habit, you'll find that your blemishes are diminished, fine lines are minimized, and your entire skin looks alive and refreshed. It's like taking a shower on the inside.

A healthy diet of fruits, vegetables, and lean proteins will not only help the way you look. It will also increase your energy levels dramatically while enhancing your natural beauty. Balance is the key here, so I discourage diets. They create a sense of deprivation which inevitably results in obsessive overeating. This wreaks havoc on the system, and the skin is the first place to show the inner chaos. Women on diets generally complain to me that their skin breaks out, or it gets dry and laced with fine lines. This is the body's natural reaction to unpredictable nourishment, as it struggles to stabilize under difficult and constantly changing conditions.

RELAXING THE MIND AND BODY

Sleep, although crucial to your health, is not the same as relaxation. Getting manicures, pedicures, facials, and massages are the ultimate form of pampering. When I leave a spa after receiving any of these wonderful treatments, I always feel renewed. I've never met a woman who didn't like some form of massage, as the healing touch works wonders for stress release and sore muscles. Treatments such as the ones listed can quiet the mind, make you feel better about yourself, and help you cope with the daily stresses we all have in our busy lives.

There are so many ways to create relaxation in your life. Go to the park when the kids are in school and read a book. Schedule it in as you would a business meeting. If you work all day and can't take the luxury of visiting a park, take a bath filled with aromatherapy or chamomile bath salts before you go to bed. If you can't afford a massage or a manicure, get together with a group of friends and hire someone to come to

Xini and me

your home to work on all of you. Women often look to their husbands and boyfriends for nurturing, but nine times out of ten, bonding with your women friends for pampering and beauty treatments will give you much better results.

HELPFUL HINTS:

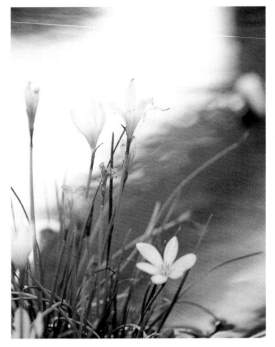

- Do your exercise at the same time every day. You'll have a better chance of sticking to your routine.

- Think of exercise as a way of life. Take the stairs instead of the elevator, do sit-ups while you watch TV, and stretch often throughout the day.

- Flexibility equals youthfulness.

- Drinking lots of water will diminish blemishes, minimize fine lines, and make your skin glow.

BEAUTY MARK

1:

Choose a form of exercise you like to ensure sticking with it.

BEAUTY MARK

2:

Maintaining a stable weight and drinking water preserves your skin's natural elasticity.

Who would you rather be—a skinny woman who throws up her food after every meal and feels terrible, or a healthy woman of average weight, who feels happy to be alive? The answer seems obvious, but there are so many women suffering with anorexia and bulimia these days, and no amount of money can help them buy their way out of it. Personally, I've been broke and I've had money, and neither of these two states assured me misery or happiness.

Since we're living so much longer now, health must be our number one concern. Yet, statistics don't seem to reflect this, even as we find out that overly skinny women are more prone to osteoporosis, that bulimia eats away not only your stomach lining, but also the enamel on your teeth. Young girls are still trying to fashion themselves after waifs and supermodels. The fact that Kate Moss ended up in rehab last year seems to have no bearing on their decisions.

The important point here is that we are all different. Some of us were born to be slim, while others are far more healthy with a few extra pounds on our frames. We need to love our reflection in the mirror as we are, and then, if we think losing a few pounds will make us feel better, there are healthy ways to accomplish that with sensible food and exercise. Let's drop the misconception that skeletons are sexy (men don't think so), and embrace our own health and beauty, exactly as we are.

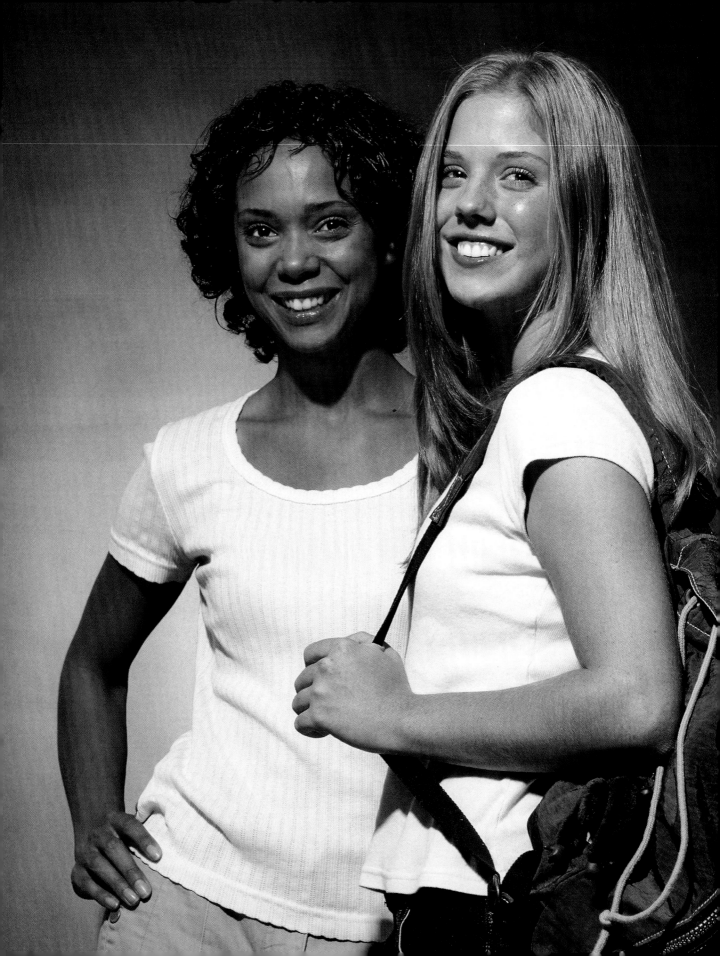

16: COMING OF AGE: TEENS & MAKEUP

WHEN DO YOU BEGIN? It's difficult to determine the right age for a teenager to start using makeup. When you walk through a fashion mall, you see a variety of cutting edge cosmetic lines popping up for teens, like Hard Candy and Urban Decay. "Generation X" makeup, which concentrates on funky, avant-garde colors that appeal to teens, has become big business, as it's gone from nail polish to mainstream cosmetics in a stunningly short period of time. Even Calvin Klein has come out with a teenage makeup line that features bright colors and promotes risk-taking attitudes. And why not? It's good business. Whether or not it's always good for teens, though, is another story. Who's more susceptible to suggestion and peer pressure than teenagers who love to cruise the malls? They want to look and act like models and rock stars. They want to be accepted. Since they don't yet know who they are, they copy what they see.

When I see my teenage son Evan's friends, I'm fascinated that some of the teenage girls are eager to use makeup at a very young age, while others just don't seem to care. For the majority, it's simply about belonging. I have a niece who started wearing a little bit of lipstick when she was ten. Although that sounds young, she always looked tasteful. Her mother allowed her to increase her makeup in very small degrees year by year, but she always kept it in check, and she never overdid it.

This is in keeping with my philosophy not to deny your teenager makeup, but to control it. You know the routine—how kids rush toward anything that's forbidden. You were a teen yourself, remember? The truth is your daughter is going to find a way to get hold of that tube of lipstick one way or the other, whether she sneaks yours, uses her friend's, or buys one at the mall or the drugstore. Teens are desperately trying to find ways to define themselves, so why not give your daughter permission to use makeup and some good guidance at the same time?

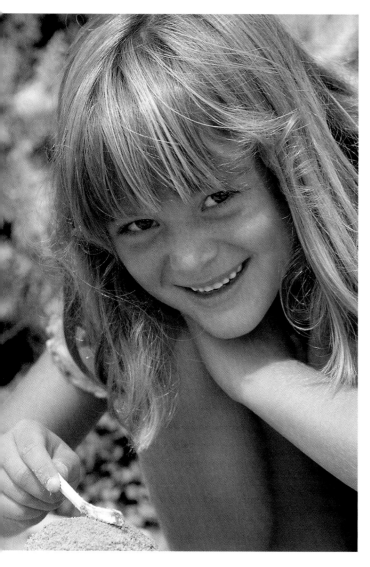

Sweet Ali

A LITTLE GOES A LONG WAY
My six-year-old daughter, Ali, loves to play with makeup. In fact, she started when she was four, running into my room and asking me to put some color on her tiny lips. Little girls spend so much time watching their mothers do their faces for work or for special events, makeup represents a coming of age. I remember when I was a teenager that I could hardly wait to shave my legs. I found a razor once, snuck into the bathroom, and shaved my legs for the first time, cutting them all up. This is typical behavior for teenagers who are so anxious to grow up and do the things they see their mothers do.

The teen years are far from easy. During this challenging time, everything about us is changing. We feel out of control so much of the time, our hormones are on overdrive, our skin gets oily, and we're moving too fast to stop and do much about it. We know so little about ourselves as individuals that discovering our best facial features is barely the tip of the iceberg. Teens are striving for answers to deeper questions like: Who am I? What do I like? What's cool and what isn't?

In the midst of such a powerful time of self-discovery and an overwhelming urge to fit in, it's important to start teenagers out with the right information. I'm pleased when mothers ask me to show their daughters how to use makeup, because it's an opportunity to train them right out of the gate. My goal with teens is to encourage them to use makeup subtly, not to hide behind it, but rather to use it in discovering and expressing their individual identities. The best makeup advice I can give teens is that a little goes a long way.

TEENAGE MAKEUP APPLICATION
Skin care is essential for teens, not only to keep your skin clean and feeling good, but to establish healthy patterns that will serve you well for the rest of your life. Be sure to wash your face both morning and night. If you wear makeup, get in the habit of always removing it before you go to sleep. If your skin is oily and it tends to break out, be extra careful to clean it well and use cleansing products and moisturizers that are oil-free.

For teen makeup application:

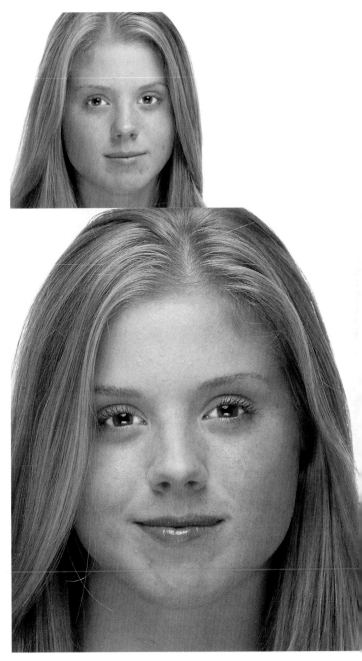

- Spot your face with a cream foundation that is very sheer, only where it's needed. You'll be amazed at what a few little dots and dabs can do.

- Your brows are thick and luxurious in your teens. You probably won't need to use eyebrow pencil and please use restraint in tweezing. It takes time to perfect shaping your brows, and a thin brow will look unnatural.

181

- I designed a dual mascara wand especially for teenagers that's clear on one side. This will give the illusion of thickening and building the lashes without adding the intensity of dark color. If you want some color, go lightly with brown over your lashes and make sure to comb through any clumps.

- Play with shimmery shadows and blushes. Remember to use a light touch.

- Have fun with lipstick shades and glosses. Red usually ends up looking too severe, so try my peaches and pinks instead.

If you want to toss a few items in your backpack (check with your parents and school rules concerning makeup), include a sheer lipstick or gloss, a little blush, and a brown or clear mascara.

MAKING MISTAKES

When you're a teenager, it's the perfect time for makeup mistakes. I encourage you to have some fun in the middle of this intense time of figuring it all out, so be bold and playful with your makeup. It all washes off at the end of the day, so why make it so serious? Instead of carefully following a trend that works for someone else, makeup can help you find your own style and create the message you want to put out. After all, everyone is different, and if you don't experiment and make a few mistakes along the way, you'll never find out what works and what doesn't.

I've been distressed at the heavy-handed made-up look that some of the magazines are showing for teenagers. And yet, I'm happy to say that a few of the current teen magazines, have begun presenting their young models in much more subtle,

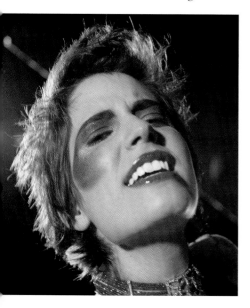

fresh-looking ways. There's a lot of room to play with cosmetics and still be subtle, and I encourage teenagers to use makeup as an outlet for their creativity.

Since you look to your friends for validation and advice, why not get together with your girlfriends and play with different looks and colors? You can make all your mistakes together, have a good time while you're at it, and when you wash it off and go home, you just may have learned something new about yourself. I read an article in a magazine recently in which a young girl picked out an outfit for herself that she thought represented who she was. Then her friends picked out an outfit for her. The result was that her friends viewed her in a very different way than she did. By listening to what they had to say and trying out their suggestions, she expanded her view of herself.

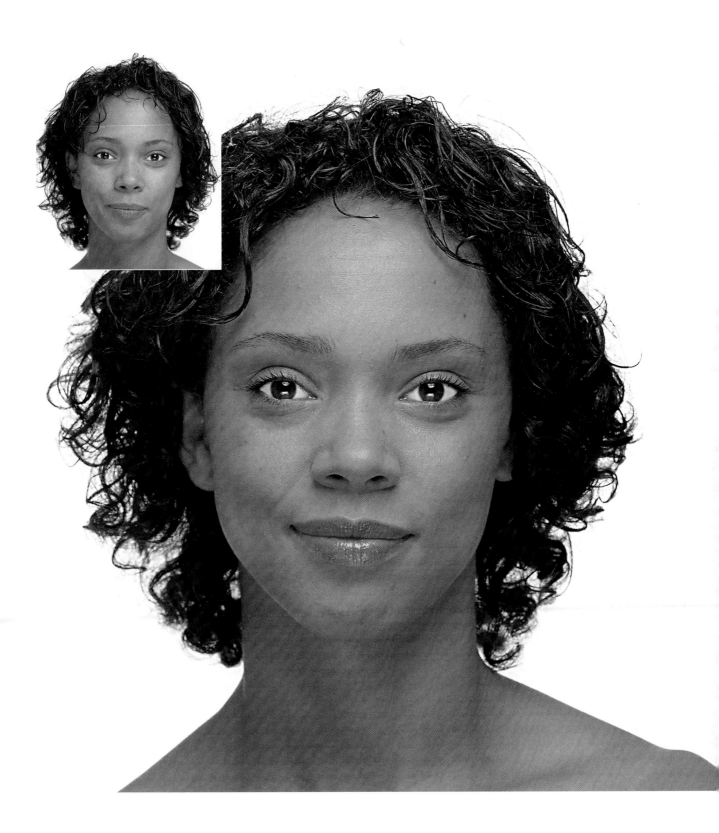

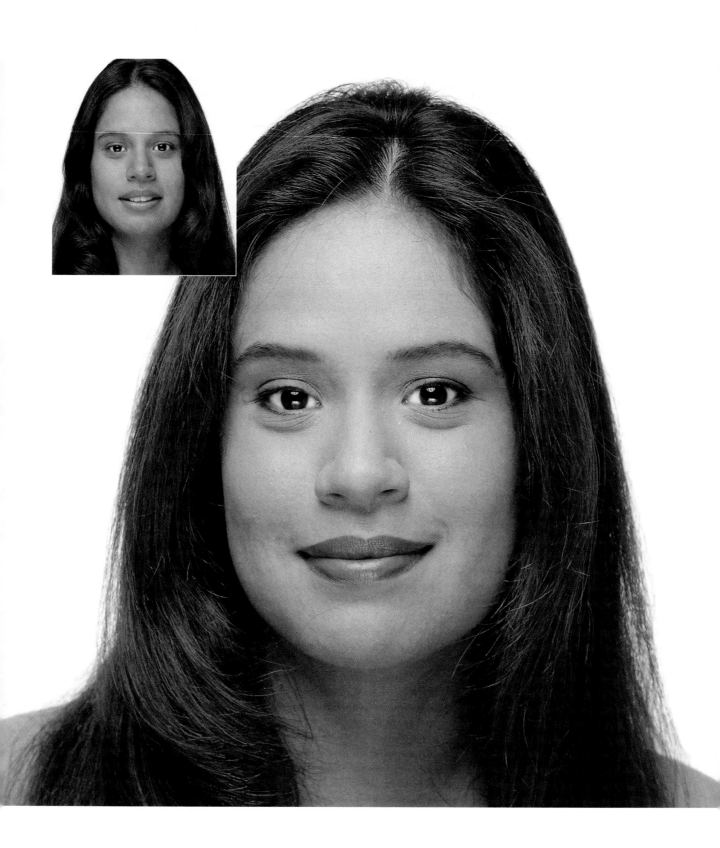

PROM NIGHT During all the excitement, it's easy to overcompensate and put on too much makeup. I encourage you to have fun with makeup on prom night, but remember that you're going to be looking at that prom photo for a long time. You want your look to be all about you, as opposed to someone you saw in a magazine or your closest friend.

My best advice is to practice your makeup before the event itself. You don't want to wait until the big night when you're nervous and there's just too much going on. If you play with your makeup the night before, you can experiment all you want. If you don't like it, you'll have plenty of time to wash it off and start over. Once you've figured out what looks best and makes you feel confident, you'll know how long it takes and you'll also know what steps are involved. Always give yourself some extra time so you won't feel rushed.

Here's a breakdown of a good prom night makeup from start to finish. This is the one night your parents will probably cut you a little slack, so play with your face and have fun!

- Spot apply foundation as needed. Cover your entire face if necessary, but do it with a very light touch. Heavy coverage will create too much texture. Be careful not to get any on your dress.

- Only do your brows as needed. If they need a little help, use a taupe eyebrow pencil and feather lightly.

- Use eye pencil on top lids as close to the lash line as possible and smudge. Do bottom lids very lightly if desired. This is a time you might want to try liquid eyeliner, but take care that it doesn't go on too thickly. Easy does it because you can't smudge the liquid.

- Use light brown mascara or black if you choose, clear side first and then color. Comb through for clumps.

- Key in your blush colors to blend with your dress. If you're wearing chiffon and pastels, go with very soft color. If you're wearing black or a dark color, try a little bit darker blush.

- Let your lip color blend with your dress. Glosses look great on teens.

- Try lightly sprinkling body shimmer on your arms and legs. It's a lot of fun and you'll sparkle in the dance lights.

185

Carry a Prom Purse with you for makeup touch-ups. It should contain a lipstick and a lip gloss, blush, foundation, an eye pencil, and I'd suggest waterproof mascara. You won't be crying (I hope not, anyway), but you will be dancing and perspiring. Nothing looks worse than streaks of mascara running down your cheeks and waterproof mascara is a little bit more long-lasting.

THE CHALLENGE OF ACNE

Acne can be a heartbreaking problem for teens. Just when you've finally developed an interest in the opposite sex and you want to look your best, it's as if your skin turns against you. It really doesn't matter how many adults assure you that it's normal and temporary, it's still devastating. In extreme cases, teenagers feel ashamed and want to hide in a cave until it's all over. There has to be a solution for teenagers plagued with acne that works well enough for them to feel good about themselves until they grow out of it.

Of course, the instinct is try to cover acne with heavy foundations, powders, and concealers. The problem is that more often than not, the product you're using to cover your acne and the way you're using it, is only making your condition worse. Smearing oily products over oily, broken-out skin, can create a disaster.

Since acne causes redness on the surface of the skin, the idea is to find an oil-free foundation that is yellow-based and won't aggravate the problem. There are various products on the market that will work, including mine, but you have to be very careful. Your blush needs to be oil-free as well, so don't forget to look for water-based products that won't add to your troubles. You want to cover the problem while you're healing it so when you look in the mirror, you can see beyond the acne to your natural beauty.

In my search to find a solution to this problem for teens, I ran across something that works very well. It's a kit called Proactiv, which is sold on a TV infomercial. This acne kit, created by dermatologists, is totally dedicated to the prevention and healing of teenage acne. Included is information on how to maintain a clear skin once you've found the balance. My good friend Judith Light is the spokesperson for Proactiv, and the stories that teenagers share with her are heartwarming and inspiring. This combination of products and instructions on how to use them and maintain a clear skin has changed the lives of a lot of kids who were afraid to go out on a date, or even to leave the house. If acne is your problem, I want to encourage you to call this number and give it a try. What do you have to lose?

For Proactiv, call QVC: 1 800 345-1515

HELPFUL HINTS:

- Oil-based products will aggravate teenage acne.

- Practice your makeup for special events the night before.

- For prom night, try sprinkling body shimmer on your arms and legs.

- For prom night, don't let your blush overpower your dress.

- Dark lipstick draws attention to lips. Use light colors if you have braces.

BEAUTY MARK

1:

Since 80% of sun damage happens to your skin before you turn twenty, use a good sunblock, preferably with an SPF of 20. Sunburn after sunburn will cause damage to the point where later, you'll be susceptible to skin cancers and leathery-looking skin.

BEAUTY MARK

2:

Bacteria on used washcloths can cause your skin to break out. Take a fresh washcloth each time you cleanse.

BEAUTY MARK

3:

When you can't wash your face and it gets shiny, use a mild astringent pad that you can carry in your purse.

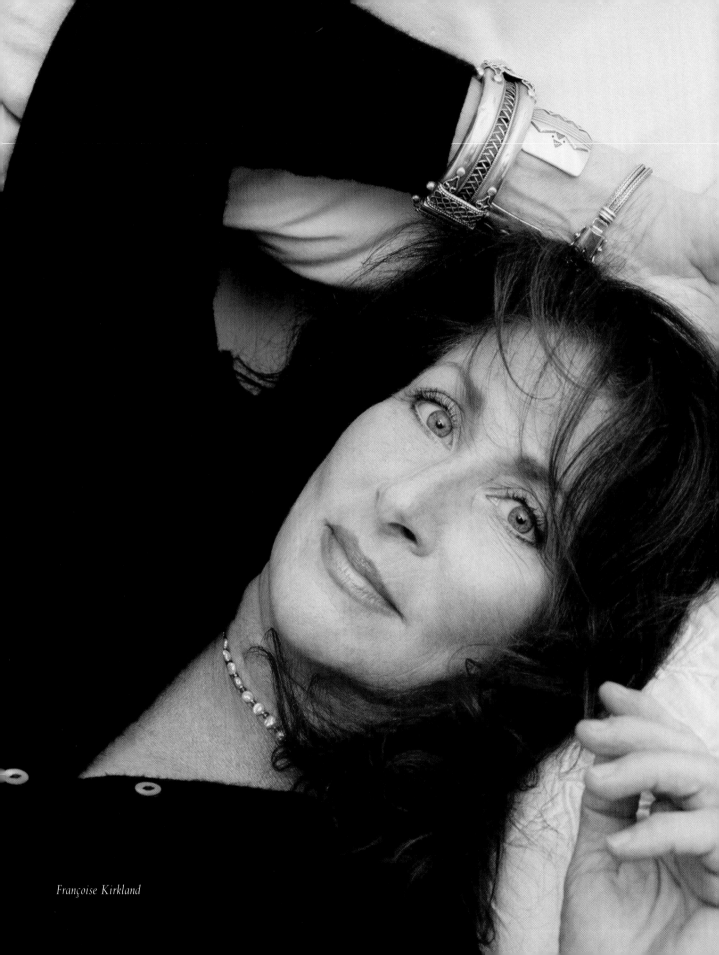

Françoise Kirkland

17: AGING: GETTING BETTER ALL THE TIME

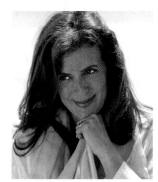

FIT AND FABULOUS Have you ever looked at an older woman who exuded so much self-confidence, you wondered how she did it? Now, all of a sudden, it seems, you're older and you realize that woman is you. Maybe you feel pretty good about yourself these days. You've finally come to understand that maturity doesn't mean you have to know everything. You've just been around a lot longer, and many of your emerging life situations are not so new and frightening. Rather, the difficulties are often reruns and you can make informed decisions based on past experience. You are no longer driven by false expectations, which greatly reduces stress. You can finally be someone who helps other women by sharing your own experiences, and there's a great comfort and sense of purpose in that. It's a terrific feeling to know a few things and to be able to give something back.

The joys and challenges of discovering who we are is a lifelong pursuit and the older I get, the more interesting it becomes. These days, our forties and fifties can be a time of core radiance and vibrancy. We can be strong, free thinking, and extremely sexy. I don't know about you, but as I continue to grow and learn, I truly feel that I'm getting better all the time.

Today, there are more women turning fifty at one time than ever before. In a certain way, it almost feels as if we're reverting back to our teenage days when it comes to peer pressure and self-acceptance. Have you noticed the tendency, once again, to compare yourself to magazine images? "Do I look better or worse than other women of my age?" you ask yourself, just as you did when you were younger and deeply insecure.

The difference here is that you have so much more of yourself to fall back on. You have your life experiences, your passions, your lifelong friends and family, and a clearer sense of what is truly important in this life. You know yourself by now, you know what feels good and what doesn't, and you've based your values and appropriate boundaries on that knowledge.

The good news about aging is that there's no longer any reason to strive to alter your image to match someone else's. I urge you, in this second half of your life, not to try to live up to anyone else's perception of beauty. Strive, instead, to create your own, to express your hard-earned self-esteem, to demonstrate your individual beauty, and to cherish yourself more than ever before.

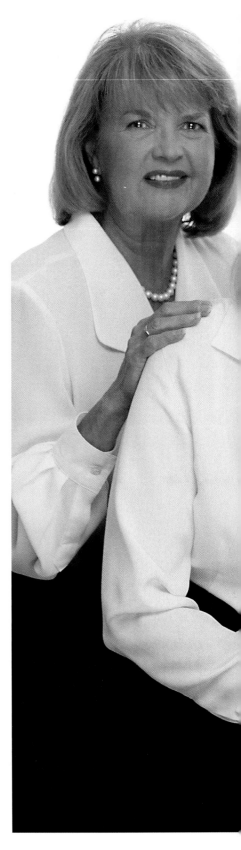

> *Character contributes to beauty. It fortifies a woman as her youth fades. A mode of conduct, a standard of courage, discipline, fortitude, and integrity can do a great deal to make a woman beautiful.*
>
> *— Jacqueline Bisset*

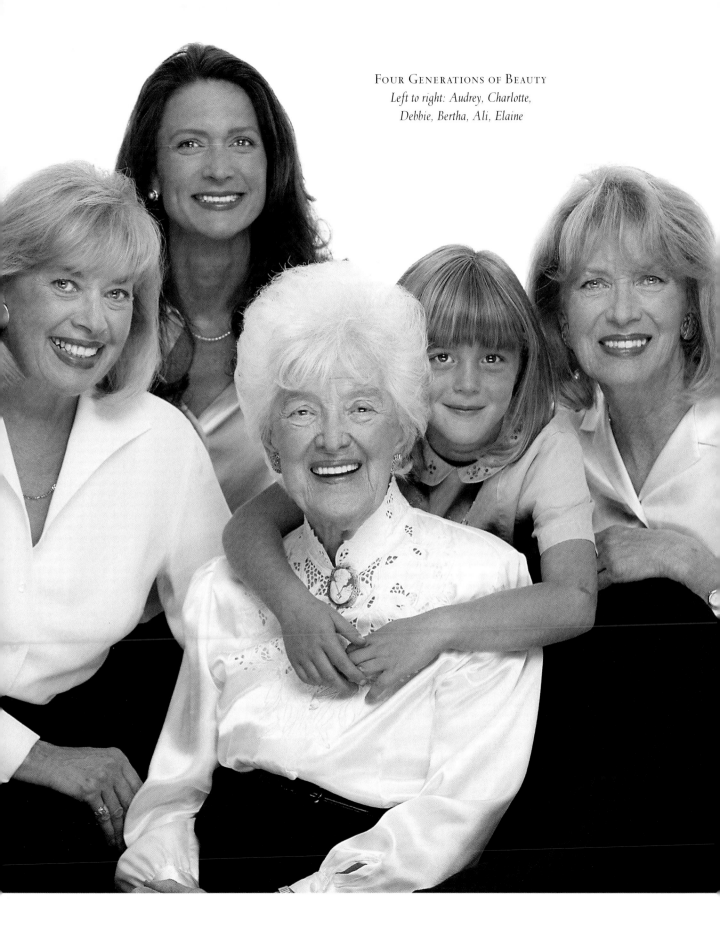

FOUR GENERATIONS OF BEAUTY
*Left to right: Audrey, Charlotte,
Debbie, Bertha, Ali, Elaine*

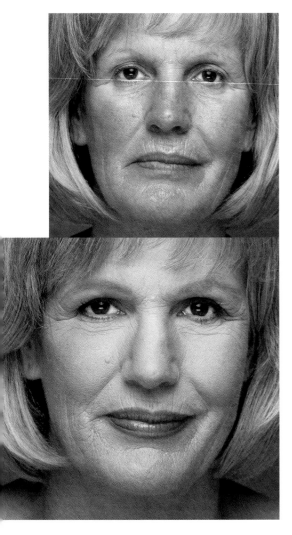

MAKEUP FOR GROWN-UPS

Let's discuss the various features of your face and how best to enhance them as you grow older. It's all in the application, in making adjustments that are in keeping with your ever-shifting beauty—like keeping your eyes open when you apply makeup, so you can see the changes in your face. Apply your makeup in an area of your home where you have plenty of light, and develop a style that really works for you NOW. Allow your clothing to reflect your growth as well. It can be fun to be a grown-up.

MOISTURIZER: Water not only improves your health but it also helps to minimize crow's feet. Drink plenty of it and make sure your moisturizer is water-based. A good one should leave your skin feeling dewy and plumped out. Then, if you need to use a little more foundation for coverage and concealing, your skin won't feel dried up underneath. Remember, the better the moisturizer, the more evenly your skin will grab makeup. Just apply it evenly and your makeup will look nice and smooth.

FOUNDATION: It's important to use a foundation that goes on smoothly and feels moist. There are products on the market that claim to be vitamin-enriched, but I'm not so convinced that it's true or that vitamins are even the answer. I still wear my own foundation, the same product I manufactured and wore in my twenties, not only because it's mine, but because it still works. I formulated it with all ages in mind, so even if I put a little bit more on my sponge, the product still works great. And I still remember to blend, blend, blend.

As I mentioned above, beware of popular cosmetic lines that formulate their makeup with teens in mind. It may have worked great for you back then, but now you need something that covers better and relates more to the type of skin changes that happen as you get a little older. Since hormonal changes can cause short flare-ups of acne, you may want to use an over-the-counter blemish cream under your foundation. Always look at the marketing concept behind the product, it's a dead giveaway, and figure out which companies are marketing cosmetics for your age group. It'll make all the difference.

If brown spots are a problem, especially if you've been a sun worshiper, first check with a doctor to make sure they aren't skin cancers. If all is well (as in most cases), a good foundation and perhaps a concealer will generally do the trick. You can also check with your dermatologist about ways to chemically lighten sun spots if they're extreme.

Here's a foundation trick for a softening of your chin line. If you notice an extra fullness at the chin, begin by improving your posture and holding your head high. For special occasions or photographs, draw a thick line of darker foundation along the jawbone with a Q-tip. Blur the line completely with a sponge, blending it over the fuller area. Call attention upward with good eye and cheek makeup.

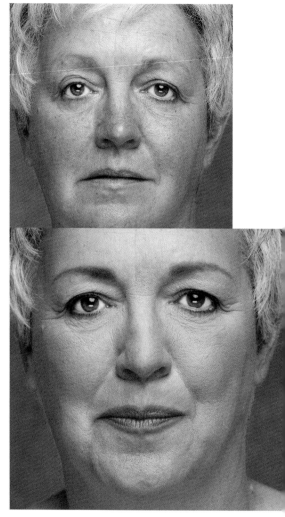

- POWDER: When I was a teen, I almost never wore powder. I still wear very little, but for you, that depends upon preference and skin type, which usually change over the years. If you've been plagued by oily skin all your life, you may be in for a big surprise. Some women find that as they mature, their skin stops breaking out, and they end up with fewer lines than women who had normal or dry skin all their lives and no acne problems. (Yes, it's a form of justice). Remember that old line, "It all comes out in the wash." It's true with your skin, so you may not need powder anymore. Keep in mind that with the exception of bronzer, powder is not for depositing color. It's for absorbing excess oils and getting rid of shine. If you don't have any, why bother using powder? If you want to use it, the current manufacturing techniques have improved and the powders are so finely milled, you'll find products that don't add texture, but rather help to diffuse light and take down shine.

- EYES: As we age, our eyebrows get more sparse. Isn't it ironic that when you finally get tweezing down, your eyebrows stop growing back? Most women's brows get sparser and lighter in their late thirties or early forties. Use my taupe eyebrow pencil to feather in your brows, being careful to blend and create a natural-looking brow to frame your face.

Eyelashes get sparser, too. If your eyelashes are gone completely due to chemotherapy or an illness, then false eyelashes are a good answer. There are new ones available called "individuals," which go on lash by lash, and look much more real than the old-fashioned type that come on a strip and are pretty thick and unnatural-looking. I don't suggest false eyelashes unless yours are completely gone, simply because the glue will end up removing whatever real lashes you may have left. Some women with sparse lashes choose to dye them, which is a safer, better solution. At least you won't be reducing what you still have.

Makeup helped me "jump-start" my life again. This fall, at seventy years old, I'll be entering the job market again, and I didn't know how to do my eyes. Knowing the right makeup techniques gave me what I needed to feel confident and look better. Isn't that wonderful?

—D.S. Detroit, MI

The most common problem for women past forty or fifty is that the eyelid tends to droop. To counteract gravity, I suggest applying your eye shadow on the outer portion of your lid and then reshaping the eye, as opposed to following the natural contours. This will create the illusion of lifting the eye. Keep in mind that iridescent and shimmer shadows will attract attention to your eyes, which may be contradictory to the illusion you're trying to create. Try using softer, more neutral brown, earthy tones. These deeper and richer hues add a certain depth, while lighter colors will flatten out the area, something you don't want to do. At the same time, key into the colors of your iris, or your clothes. Remember to hold the eye taut and manipulate the delicate skin with your hands while applying, in order to work with crevices and lines that didn't challenge you when you were in your twenties.

When you apply eyeliner, look straight in the mirror and do it with your eyes open. This will allow the liner to end up exactly where you intend it to be. I suggest pencil liner, which smudges and blends much better than other types. If you have dark shadows or circles beneath your eyes, you might want to skip the under-eye liner which tends to exaggerate the problem. If you want to line your under-eyes, a light brown pencil is your best bet. Create a broken line of color between the bottom lashes to make them look really natural.

- BLUSH: I don't suggest any dramatic shifts in blush application. Just smile and apply color on the apple of your cheeks and keep it soft.

- LIPS: Most women use lip liner when they get older. This is because our lips begin to shrink in size, and we can see fine lines developing. By the way, this happens both to thin and thick lips, so whichever you have, avoid heavy glosses which bleed into lines. Wear products that are emollient and feel dewy, not glossy or drying.

Since lips tend to lose some of their natural color as we age, lipstick can make all the difference. Just keep in mind that lip liner will help stop color from bleeding into those fine lines, and pencils will create a softer, more rounded, less severe look in their application.

GRACE AND DIGNITY

Although our numbers are larger than ever before, there's also a great deal of denial about aging among the baby boomer generation. When you were in your twenties and aging seemed so remote and unreal, it was easy to talk about growing old gracefully. Then one day, it sneaks up when you least expect it, and take it from me—this thing that was so distant is suddenly knocking on your door, staring at you in the mirror, and creating challenges that you never really believed you'd have. It isn't easy to grow old with dignity in a society that associates aging with becoming less attractive and less valuable. This couldn't be further from the truth, but the messages are pervasive. It takes a strong woman to defy popular myths and programming. How can so many of us be in so much denial? How can we age gracefully, demonstrating dignity and character to a world that encourages us to lie about our ages?

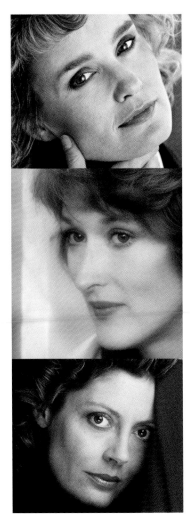

I challenge women, here and now, to find ways to feel good about getting older, to radiate their beauty, and to place dignity and grace in these previously forbidden realms, so we can all relax into this potentially rewarding phase of life. It's up to us.

For starters, we need to talk honestly about lines and wrinkles. We all get them eventually, and contrary to what many people seem to think, they're not necessarily a bad thing. Think about great beauties like Meryl Streep, Jessica Lange, Helen Hayes, and Jessica Tandy who never lost their appeal. Keep in mind that crow's feet and other fine lines are the result of smiling and laughing over a lifetime, so they can't be all bad.

I want to make it quite clear here that I'm not suggesting there's nothing you can do with makeup to minimize wrinkles and still retain character. Of course, there is. I just want to suggest that we can all work to make some strides in accepting ourselves as we are. Then, when we make up our faces, we'll be less inclined to overdo it and more inclined to accentuate our gifts.

Makeup can be your friend during this time, not only to conceal, but as ever, to enhance your natural beauty. Remember that covering lines and wrinkles can be a tricky proposition, so you need to take your time and know what you're doing. The concentration as we age needs to be on lifting everything upward (think north), because your eyelids, your eyes, and your skin, tend to droop as you get older. Softening and blending are the focus here, rather than contrast and texture. You want to create an evenness to your skin in order get a really good coverage for your lines, while you avoid adding texture, which often accentuates what you're trying to minimize. I'm not advising you suddenly to become timid. There's no need to think that your days of playful, fabulous makeup are over. The advantage here is that the older you are, the better you know yourself. Women over forty no longer need to impress anybody because their instincts are well-grounded and dependable.

If you're one of us, expressing yourself should be getting easier all the time, so relax into it and enjoy playing with makeup. Just keep your expectations realistic, keep your eyes open, and you'll do fine. The days of snake oil are over, so forget the old "hope in a jar" routine. You've got plenty of hope in your heart by now, so be real, playful, and expressive. Why should you try to make yourself look twenty when you're fifty? Keep evolving and go for something new.

BEAUTY MARK

1:

To avoid color from bleeding and to erase fine lines around lips, dip tip of lip brush into foundation and lightly outline lips.

BEAUTY MARK

2:

Lip liner will help eliminate color bleeding into fine lines.

BEAUTY MARK

3:

An improved posture will de-emphasize fullness in the chin area.

BEAUTY MARK

4:

Too much powder will add texture that emphasizes lines and wrinkles.

- If you're concerned with lines and wrinkles, go easy on shimmer and iridescent shadows as they accentuate lines and wrinkles.

- When applying foundation and powder, cover skin fully, but keep it sheer enough to avoid texture which accentuates wrinkles and lines.

- Create a broken line of light color between the bottom lashes to make under-eye liner look natural.

- Drinking water naturally reduces crow's feet.

- Brown spots could be indicators of skin cancer, so be sure to consult with a doctor if you have any concerns.

- Lip pencils make it easy to create a soft, rounded look.

MYTH:

YOUTH EQUALS BEAUTY

REALITY:

BEAUTY IS TIMELESS

We all hear about ageless, timeless beauty, but do you really believe it exists? I don't know about you, but I've seen women in their forties and fifties whose beauty takes my breath away. Think about Rene Russo in *The Thomas Crown Affair*. She's forty-four with children, and people around the world were talking about how amazing she looked.

How many times have we been told that men get better with age, but women don't? Maybe your face at fifty isn't as smooth or peaches and creamy as it once was, but what about the character and the wisdom that shines through an older woman's eyes? The more women stop trying to disguise their ages, the more we will be appreciated at every age. Be proud of your face and your experiences. Walk tall no matter your years, stop lying about your age, and your beauty will be recognized and celebrated by everyone. It all begins with you.

AGING: GETTING BETTER ALL THE TIME

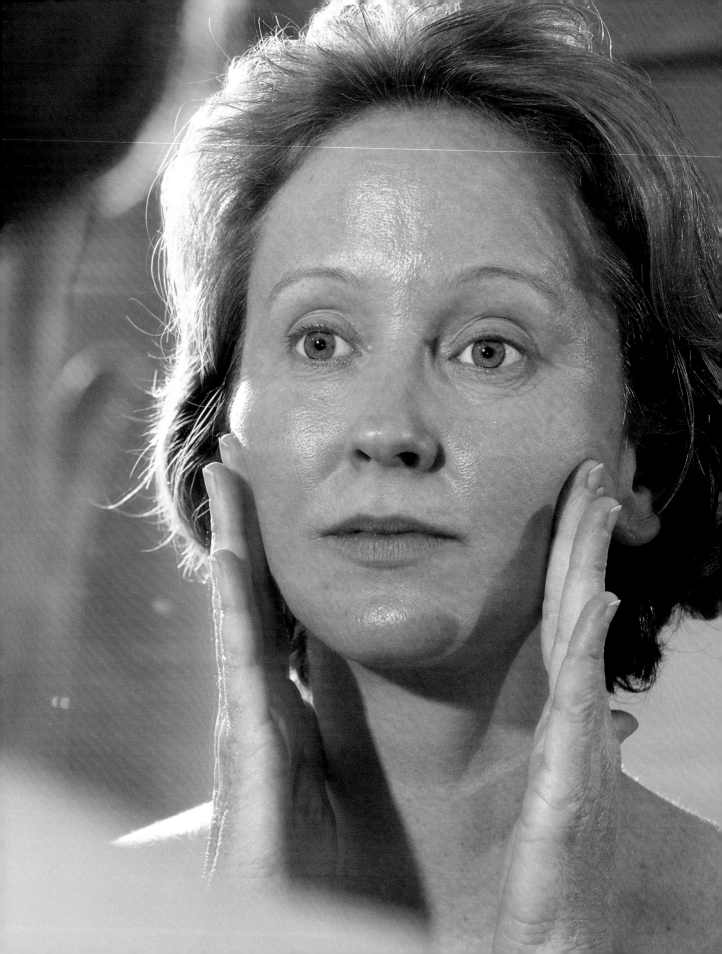

18: PLASTIC SURGERY: THE DOUBLE-EDGED SWORD

THE BIG DILEMMA Everybody's doing it. Or so it seems. *Newsweek* reports that while the number of reconstructive surgeries for emergencies like lacerations and burns have remained fairly stable over the years, cosmetic enhancements have risen dramatically. According to a new report by the American Society of Plastic and Reconstructive Surgery, cosmetic procedures have increased by 153 percent since 1992, reaching a whopping number in excess of one million during 1998. This excludes the enormous amount of work done by noncertified specialists such as dermatologists, dentists (you figure it), and gynecologists. The June, 1999, edition of *McCall's* magazine says that out of 500 women surveyed, fifty-seven percent said they would opt to go under the knife if plastic surgery were both affordable and totally safe. Twenty-six percent chose eyes as the most lusted-after surgery, while eighteen percent wanted breast enhancements.

The truth is that neither affordability nor safety are as yet assured, so while plastic surgery can be a great gift, it can also be the booby prize. When you consider the possible successes, failures, and all that come in between, you understand that cosmetic surgery can be your friend or it can turn on you, giving you a lot more than you bargained for. It's crucial to take the time to do adequate research, so you'll know what you're doing and whom you're hiring for such a serious alteration of your precious body. Making informed decisions is most of the battle. The part that's left is all about attitude with a little bit of luck thrown in.

If you have a feature that's really bothering you, like a bump on your nose or bags under your eyes, and no amount of makeup can cover it or distract from it, try to make peace with it. If you can't, plastic surgery may be the way to go. I urge you, before you make any permanent changes on your face or body, to ask yourself the following questions:

- Who are you doing this for? Your boyfriend, your husband, your boss, your girlfriends, or yourself?

- Do you expect to receive more love from other people after you change that feature on your face?

- How is your self-esteem? Are you trying to create an inner shift by altering the outside? That doesn't work.

- Have you done enough realistic research to know whether or not your expectations are too high? Are you trying to look like Cindy Crawford or a better version of you?

- Do you know the doctor you've chosen well enough to discern his expertise? Do you know his past and have you seen his work on others or are you just taking his or somebody else's word for it?

- Did you choose your doctor based on saving money? This isn't like finding the best deal on a new stereo. It's your face.

- Are you willing and able to take the appropriate amount of time to heal properly?

- Do you have the patience to wait for the results to show up?

These are all important questions to ask yourself before you go forward with a procedure from which there's no turning back. I faced these questions myself when I was unhappy with the excess fatty tissue under my eyes. I had just turned forty-one, and I knew all the makeup tips for bags under the eyes. For years, I'd taken my liner and applied it low enough into my lash line to create the illusion of cutting the puffy parts in two, all to no avail. No matter how hard I tried and how much time I took, I couldn't disguise them. I finally realized that a puff is a puff is a puff. There was really nothing I could do except live with them or have them surgically removed. Since I'm in the beauty business and everyone looks at my face through a microscope, it really bothered me.

I took the leap, but not until I did a ton of research. After all, I was about to have a scalpel cutting around my eyeballs, which is a very scary thing to consider. I'd heard horror stories and seen enough bad results to take a great deal of time to make my final decision. When I found a doctor whom I initially liked and felt I could trust, I asked to see his previous work, both in photographs and on real people. I liked what I saw. Then, I got completely educated on what could go wrong, what the chances were of being disappointed, and what the healing process involved. I wanted to know my part in it, how I could affect my own healing in a positive way.

CHASING BARBIE
Then the next phase of my work began. I looked inside to see who I was really doing this for. I knew that under-eye surgery wouldn't make me feel better about who I was on the inside or make anyone else love me more. When I determined that I wanted to do this solely for me and for my business, I made the decision to proceed.

I remember immediately after the operation, the nurse came to me with a mirror. She wanted me to see my eyes before they swelled up. "Take a look at yourself before it looks like a truck hit you," she said. I appreciated that. I kept my attitude positive, I ate well and slept a lot, and I healed quickly with no complications. Today, several years later, I'm happy with the results. For me, the best part was and still is that I no longer have to take the time and effort each day to cover my under-eye bags. I can put that one behind me now.

I like to think that my good experience was due to research, attitude, and realistic expectations. I've met too many women who were chasing after the Barbie Doll image, either hunting for perpetual youth or trying to look different from what they are. The truth is that cosmetic surgery is much more prevalent in places like New York, Los Angeles, and Dallas because unrealistic expectations are higher in these cosmopolitan cities. We seem to create pressure to look a certain way and not to age in the bigger cities. In more rural communities, the standards about women's looks are not so crazy and women are far less competitive. We could take a few lessons from them.

PLASTIC FANTASTIC
I'm sorry to even have to address the topic of plastic surgery for teens, but the reality is shocking. There are larger and larger numbers of teenagers having plastic surgery and liposuction done on everything from their breasts to their lips, from their thighs to their eyes. I can't imagine how a doctor in his right mind could perform these kinds of serious operations on teenagers,

but the sad truth is that they do it all the time. *Newsweek*, August 9, 1999, reports that in 1998, 1,645 patients eighteen years of age and younger had liposuction, while 1,840 had their breasts enlarged. This was twice as many as in 1992, so the trend is clearly on the rise.

Since I don't like to speak in absolutes, I have to say that there are certain exceptions to the "no teen plastic surgery" rule, for example noses or body features that create physical problems. Many teenage girls have their noses done. Although I still see the wisdom in waiting until they mature, a nose will pretty much stay the same, so there seems to be less harm there. Lips, on the other hand, are a different story. Too many teens have their lips plumped up before their facial structures are fully developed. We all know the trouble with breast implants, a danger which has spoken loudly enough for itself over the past couple of decades. Until a woman is old enough to understand the implications of losing the ability to breast feed and can view her body image in a mature way, I strongly urge her to wait to make such serious, life-changing, potentially dangerous decisions.

ALTERNATIVE FACIAL PROCEDURES
Surgery is not the only answer to facial alterations. There are some wonderful technological breakthroughs these days that can help you create a beautiful face without losing your character. Some of these nonsurgical, noninvasive methods are less extreme than others. In fact, there are several you can do on your lunch hour. Once again, take all the pros and cons into consideration before you act because there are consequences and risks with all procedures, and sometimes the far-reaching effects negatively outweigh the positive ones. Keep your eyes and ears open, know what you're getting into, and make your decisions from an informed place. The good news is that many dermatologists can do one or more of these alternative procedures in her office, while others will require a specialized surgeon and a hospital-like setting.

BOTOX: A doctor injects a Botulism poison (sorry, that's what it is) into your facial muscles which temporarily paralyzes them. You are asked to lie down for a few hours after the treatment to avoid the substance from traveling beneath the skin to other areas of the face. This treatment was originally created to inhibit spasms and facial tics, but it was also found to inhibit the involuntary facial contractions that cause wrinkles, a furrowed brow, and crow's feet.

You'll feel a minimal pin prick from the injection, followed by a mild burning sensation that leaves quickly. It takes about a week to experience the full results, and the positive effects eventually wear off in about four months when they need to be repeated. Doctors report an additional benefit—when the Botox wears away, the original lines and furrows are less deep due to the lack of facial contractions over an extended period of time.

Take Care: Potential problems are drooping eyelids if the insertion point is done too close to the eye. If too many injections are administered at once, your natural facial expressions can be arrested.

COLLAGEN INJECTIONS: This collagen, useful in recessing scars, filling in facial creases, and plumping up wrinkles, is derived from cow skin. A doctor can safely inject several facial areas in one session, such as the forehead, the cheeks, and the smile lines. The typical lasting time is four to six months, after which the substance will gradually deflate over a few months because the body is programmed to break it down.

The pain is generally mild, some areas tending to be more difficult than others. A topical agent will lessen the pain, and it will take a few hours to a few days for your skin to lose redness and tenderness. With lips, swelling and soreness can last two to three days.

Take Care: Always pretest this procedure as bovine collagen causes allergic reactions in sensitive people. A bad reaction, caused by the body reabsorbing the collagen too quickly, has been linked to auto-immune disorders. Bruising is possible.

FAT TRANSPLANTS: An alternative to collagen injections, a doctor uses a syringe to take living fat tissue from your thighs or buttocks and injects it into smile lines, pitted scars, or lips, There's no chance of allergic reactions because it's your own body which can easily store the fat, and it should last for up to a year. The drawback is that fat tissue is thicker than bovine fat, so precision is more difficult than with bovine collagen.

The tiny incisions cause minimal pain, and stitches are necessary. The area from which fat is removed must be wrapped to avoid indentations. Soreness and swelling in both removal and injection areas will last for about one to two days. Expect bruising.

Take Care: The tissue's ability to link with the blood supply in that area is not guaranteed, which makes longevity "iffy." The injections may need to be done repeatedly until it "takes."

DERMABRASION: A doctor uses a high-speed rotary wire brush or diamond disk to sand off the top layer of skin cells. Laser procedures and light chemical peels have become more popular, but dermabrasion is sometimes recommended on areas that require extra help such as cheeks and upper lips. This is good for skin surface irregularities, deep wrinkles, acne, scars, and pockmarks.

A painless procedure (it's done under anesthetic), expect moderate discomfort afterward, which may require painkillers. Recovery includes raw skin, oozing, and redness, which is covered with a surgical dressing. Scabs fall off in ten days to two weeks, and the reddened skin underneath can be covered with makeup. All is normal once again in three to six months.

Take Care: Watch out for scars, infections, and pigment irregularities. Not recommended for dark skin, cold sores and acne can result in predisposed conditions.

LASER RESURFACING: A very popular treatment, this procedure vaporizes the top layers of skin while tightening the collagen layer underneath. The laser is computer-guided with great speed and accuracy to remove wrinkles and skin irregularities with tiny bursts of light. Easily programmed to the correct depth without disturbing top layers, this procedure is highly favored over dermabrasion. Laser resurfacing encourages the natural collagen to reorganize itself in a smooth fashion, to eliminate superficial wrinkles, smooth out pigmentation and skin texture, minimize scars, and resurface spots around the eyes and mouth. On certain areas, the laser can also be used for several passes in a free-hand fashion, the doctor manually wiping away vaporized skin in between. The more extensive laser procedures must be done in a hospital-like setting, a full face taking about an hour.

You may feel a slight snapping sensation, but the pain is minimal, and anesthesia is usually administered. Painkillers are recommended for post-procedure discomfort. Light resurfacing will take about a week or two to heal. Deeper work will result in redness, swelling, and oozing, and a dressing is applied. The skin crusts and flakes off from one to four months, and makeup can be used to cover after the skin heals.

Take Care: Darker skins may result in scarring and irregular pigmentation. Cold sores and acne can result in predisposed conditions.

LASER REMOVAL: This works well with pigmentation problems such as age spots, tattoos, spider veins, broken capillaries, and birthmarks. The laser emits a wavelength of light, which seeks out a certain skin color. When it finds what it's looking for, the energy begins to pulverize. The surrounding skin remains unaffected, while the targeted fragments are swept away by the body's natural internal cleansing process.

Expect mild to moderate pain. A local anesthesia is recommended in some cases. With vein procedures, the skin will be pink for a few hours, and bruising is common. With pigment removal, bleeding and blistering usually occur. The skin crusts over and the scabs fall off in a week or two to reveal a smooth, pink skin.

Take Care: Watch for incomplete removal of pigment. The area may heal lighter, darker, or with a different texture than the rest of your skin.

CHEMICAL PEELS: A chemically caused controlled inflammation of the skin will cause the outer layers to shed. This will remove pigmentation irregularities, superficial wrinkles, and fine lines while encouraging new skin and natural collagen growth. The skin flakes and peels off for several days after the procedure, subsiding quickly. The end result is more elasticity and suppleness of the skin's texture.

There are several forms available, from light to aggressive, which a doctor can determine according to your skin's needs. For all peels, you must stay out of the sun for several weeks, and for the more aggressive types, constant use of sunblock is highly suggested.

AHA PEELS: To eliminate fine lines, clear up blemishes, and add a glow to your skin, a solution of glycolic acid in concentrations of thirty to seventy percent will remove the outer epidermal layers. A qualified doctor swabs it onto the skin, and a few minutes later, rinses it off with water. Most people tolerate the acid well, but physicians usually prefer to apply it over several visits, to minimize risk.

You'll feel a light sting when the solution is applied, which will diminish quickly. Expect one hour to two weeks for redness to subside, depending upon the strength of the peel. Most of the time, you can cover the area with makeup.

Take Care: It's rare but you could experience discoloration or a sunburn-like reaction.

TCA (TRICHLOROACETIC ACID) PEELS: TCA can create a mild or deep peeling effect, depending on concentration of solution. Reaching into the top levels of the dermis, the procedure takes about a half hour and can be used on various areas of the face. Slightly stronger than an AHA peel, this will eliminate deeper wrinkles and pigmentation problems on face or hands.

The pain is mild to moderate, depending upon the depth of the peel and sedation may be required. Red and swollen skin will result from the lighter technique, which should subside in about a week. Deeper peels cause swelling and oozing, the face crusts over and peels away in a week or two. Any leftover pinkness can be covered with makeup. A few weeks later, normal skin tone returns.

Take Care: If the peel goes too deep, you may experience pigmentation loss. In predisposed conditions, cold sores or acne can result.

PHENOL PEELS: This very invasive procedure (rarely done anymore) penetrates to the midlevel of the dermis. Full-face procedures require heart monitoring, but can be effective on very deep wrinkles and profound sun damage. In fact, phenol is so strong, it's sometimes used for precancerous and cancerous lesions. Sunning afterward is strictly forbidden, as phenol impairs the skin's ability to tan.

Phenol numbs the skin during application, so pain is minimal. Some people prefer sedation, anyway, and prescription painkillers are recommended after the procedure. Forty-eight hours of recovery in bed is suggested, and the skin will be red, swollen, and oozy for eight to ten days. Scabs naturally slough off in two to three weeks, and the fresh, pink skin underneath takes from three to six months to return to normal.

Take Care: People with dark skin or diabetes are recommended to stay away. This procedure can result in scarring, skin atrophies, permanent loss of pigmentation, and damage to heart, kidneys, and liver. In predisposed conditions, cold sores or acne may result.

SUPPORT SYSTEMS

For any woman, the decision to have cosmetic surgery has to be an individual one that requires time, research, maturity, and money. For starters, no one should go through it without a good support system in place. Consult with people whom you trust and see how your husband or boyfriend feels about it. Ask your girlfriends and other family members if they think it's a good idea for you. You may discover that they're willing to support you, or you may be surprised that they aren't. If you get a negative reaction from enough trusted friends, take a second look. You may not be seeing yourself clearly.

Once you've determined that you want to take the next step, you need to choose the right doctor. No impulsive decisions here, please. Don't close your eyes, open up the phone book, and see where your finger lands. For all you know, the man that fate picks out may have never performed a surgery before and you're about to be his guinea pig. Follow these guidelines:

- Ask around your community for referrals.

- Find out about his or her track record.

- Is he or she certified? According to the August 9, 1999, edition of *Newsweek*, the American Board of Plastic Surgery requires a five year surgical residency.

- Has he or she applied to a hospital's review board for surgical privileges? If not, *Newsweek* warns, the doctor may not have his or her credentials up to snuff.

If the doctor you've chosen seems to be "iffy" in any way, move on to another. There are enough of them out there. When you've established someone who can be trusted, make sure to see her previous work, both her portfolio and some people she's done. If you like what you see, you're probably on the right track. If you have a gut feeling that something isn't quite right, don't second-guess yourself. You need to trust your instincts here, so walk away. One of the doctors I went to see had drawn women's faces all over his waiting room walls. I didn't like what I saw, so I figured if I didn't like his two-dimensional art work, I probably wouldn't like the way he did cutouts, either. Needless to say, I left. It's odd how three different doctors will give you three different opinions about your face. I met with one doctor who wasn't happy with just doing my eyes. He began rattling off a laundry list of my other features he thought were imperfect, and how he wanted to change them. I left his office feeling terrible about myself, but I learned a lot that day. I continued my search, determined that I would only have the surgery if I could walk away from the consultation with my head held high. It makes me sad to think about the number of women with no real sense of themselves who believe these kinds of doctors and have a load of unnecessary work done. When you go this route, how do you ever know when to stop? If you're twenty-five to thirty-five years old, and a doctor suggests a full face-lift and any other additional surgeries, I'd question his or her validity. This is what second, third, or even fourth opinions are for.

I want to reiterate here that finances should not be the sole determining factor. Of course, money needs to be a consideration and the better surgeons will obviously be more expensive, but if you can't afford the doctor you like, wait until you can. No bargain basement surgeons, please, because once the job is done, it's a final sale. Being in the beauty business, I've seen the best and the worst of it, and bad results are not only a heartbreak, but they can be dangerous.

That's not to say that certain mistakes can't be corrected. Surgeries often get redone with great results. At the same time, there are far too many women who go back to the cutting board over and over, and it gets worse each time. This is the ultimate plastic surgery nightmare, so do everything you can to avoid it.

A final word on plastic surgery: Plastic surgery is here to stay, and technologies are improving all the time. Do your research and give yourself a chance to have the best possible experience.

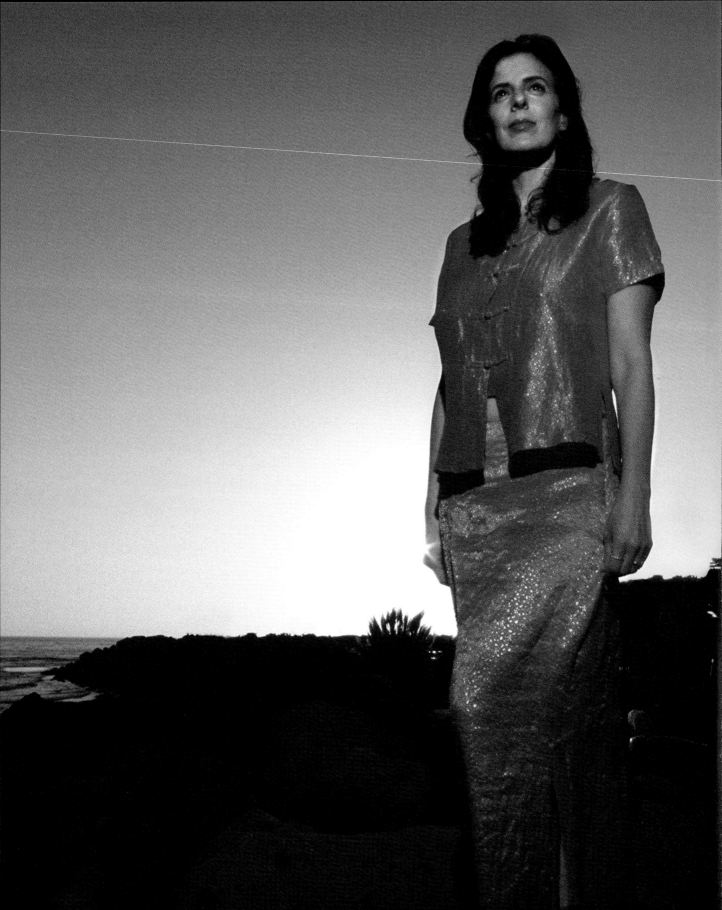

EPILOGUE

THE BOTTOM LINE Due to better education and higher self-esteem, women have gained self-confidence and a sense of entitlement about our place in the world. We no longer threaten each other in the workforce, we encourage each other instead, and we are proving to be the ultimate communicators.

One of the hardest challenges women face in modern life is balancing career and child-rearing. We really can't win on this one as yet, we get criticized for being out in the workplace, making a living, and putting the kids in day care. At the same time, we get flack if we stay home, care for the kids, and don't contribute to the family income. For you stay-at-home moms, let me acknowledge publicly that raising children full-time is harder work and takes more sacrifice than any available job in the marketplace.

The good news is that we're starting to stand up for ourselves and find solutions we can live with. We're learning to be responsible for our money, to speak up, and to be much less concerned how other people view us. We're entering all phases of business, including sports, science, medicine, and politics. No longer bound by traditional gender roles, we're not depending upon men for our survival, and we don't need their approval. As we make our own money, we're learning to stop overspending and to invest wisely.

As a result, we are finding our role models in other women, tapping into our own power to act with clarity and strength, learning to accept ourselves as we are, and allowing our curiosity and self-assurance to take us into areas where we never before dared to venture. The workplace is wide open, and instead of only acting on what is best for those around us and leaving ourselves out, we are finally asking ourselves the all-important question: "What is best for me in this situation?"

It follows that as your self-esteem increases, so will your feelings about the image you see in the mirror. Makeup is a great tool you have at your fingertips to help you accept and appreciate yourself and get on with your life, but it's only one of many. The biggest changes for women will not be external, although the outside always reflects the inside. Your knowledge of makeup and how your care for yourself in general is not about to significantly shift the way you look in the eyes of the world at large. The dramatic shifts will be in the way you feel—about yourself, your family, and your contribution to the community in which you live. Women are learning to define beauty by their own standards, not by those of men or anyone else, for that matter.

The bottom line for makeup is that technology is so far advanced from where it was, we're getting better products all around. Powders were never so sheer, lipsticks were never so creamy or long-lasting, shimmer has redefined iridescence, and the color palettes are nothing short of magnificent. Mascara, one of the most popular makeup items in the marketplace, is being made from greatly improved formulas with such fine brushes that it goes on, stays on, and creates a better effect than ever before. Makeup choices abound, so whether you wear a lot or a little, there is something really wonderful for everybody.

Women continue to get smarter, stronger, and more connected to ourselves. All this adds up to beautiful, sensual women doing business, raising families, and finding happiness with men and without them. We're making up our own lives, and in so doing, we're making the world a treasure chest of hope and opportunity for the generations to follow. Let's all keep up the good work, look fabulous, kick some butt, and have some fun along the way. I'll see you in the spotlight.

P. S.: You can write to me at:

8205 Santa Monica Boulevard, #1-210
Los Angeles, CA 90046.

For more information about my line, you can call QVC toll-free at 1-800-345-1515 or check the QVC website at http//www.QVC.com.

I'd love you to try my products, but you can follow the application steps in this book with any brand of makeup you prefer.

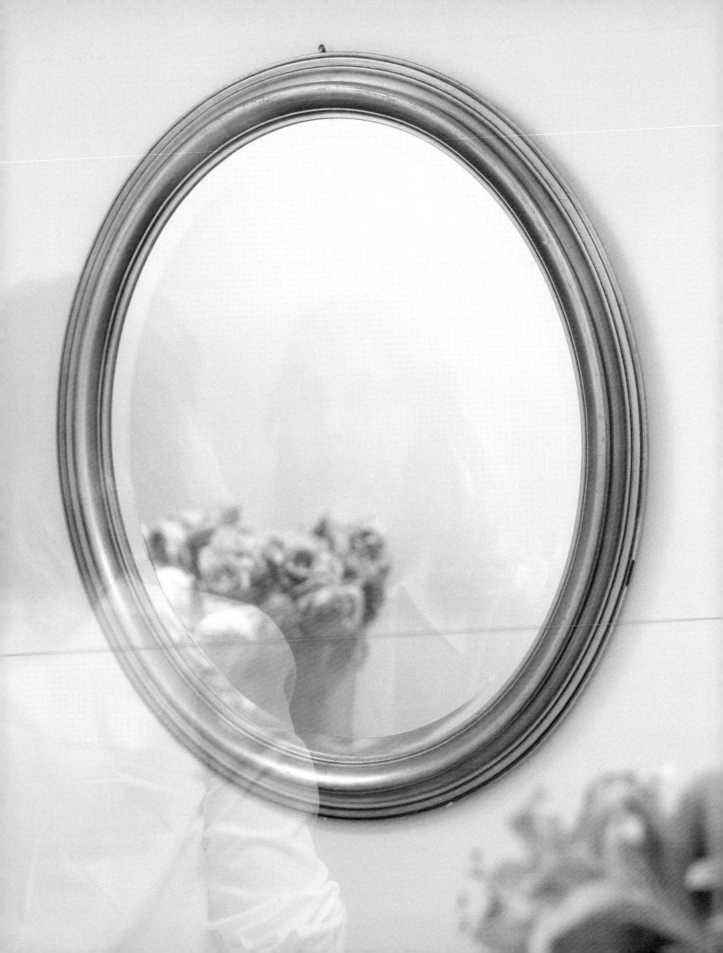

GLOSSARY

Alpha- and beta-hydroxy acids (AHAs/BHAs). Skin exfoliation agents made from fruit acids. Molecules vary in size depending on type. Generally, the smaller the molecule the more beneficial the acid. Glycolic acid falls in this category.

Antioxidants. A class of nutrients capable of preventing damage to tissues by free radicals and harmful oxidation in the body. Vitamins A, C, and E are antioxidants that are often used in skin care products.

Apple. The fleshy mound above the cheekbone that pillows up when a person smiles. It may be highlighted with a lighter shade of blush.

Astringent. A liquid or gel used primarily on oily skin to contract the pores.

Black-tie bag. Cosmetics assembled to take to a formal event for makeup touch-ups during the evening.

Blush. Pigments that add color and highlighting (or glow) to the face. Blush is available in powder, cream, or gel form.

Breakout shine. Skin oils that seep through foundation during the day and give a shiny appearance to the skin. Oil-controlling powders or oil-absorbing paper help eliminate this problem.

Bronzer. Pigment in warm tones of brown to simulate a tan or to use in place of blush on tanned skin.

Close-set eyes. A term used to describe eyes with very little space between their inner corners and the bridge of the nose.

Concealer. A special type of foundation formulated to hide complexion flaws, such as discoloration, acne blemishes, or under-eye circles. Colors range from blue to yellow or natural beige. Concealer is available in liquid, cream, or stick form.

Deep-set eyes. A term used to describe eyes that recede in the face because of prominent brows or cheekbones, and/or in which little or no lid shows when the eyes are open.

Demarcation line. A line on the skin caused by a contrast in colors that can occur when foundations or blushes are applied without blending. When referring to foundation, the demarcation line commonly occurs between the face and neck, or when facial foundation stops abruptly at the jawline. The result is a masklike appearance.

Exfoliation. The removal of the top layer of the dermis, or skin. In beauty care, this is done to stimulate the formation of new skin cells and give the skin a fresh appearance. Commonly used exfoliants are facial scrubs and loofah sponges as well as chemical agents such as alpha hydroxy lotions, cleansers, masks, and peels.

Eyebrow pencil. A makeup pencil (wooden or mechanical) containing colored pigments used to create shape and fullness to the brows. Victoria Jackson prefers taupe for fair skins, browns for darker skins. Black is not recommended; it looks unnatural.

Eyeliner. Brown or black pigments (other colors are occasionally used) applied along the edge of the upper lid above the lashes, and along the lower lid under the lashes. Liner applied on the rim of lower lid will "close down" the eye, making it look smaller. A broken line under the lower lash softens the look on aging skin. Eyeliner comes in liquid, cake, or pencil form.

Eye shadow. Colored pigments applied to the upper lid to create shadow and depth. Colors can complement eye color, hair color, or clothes. Glitters and shimmers, containing mica, may be used for dramatic events. Eye shadows come in powder or cream.

Foundation. The basic makeup applied to the skin. Its purpose is to even out the complexion and create a flawless base for the application of blush, bronzer, and powders. Foundation is available in several forms:

water-based liquid, oil-free liquid, powder-formulated, tinted moisturizer, cream, pancake or stick. A cream foundation, oil-free and sheer, applied with a sponge is preferred by Victoria Jackson. Foundation makeup, in a natural-appearing yellow base, was the first product created in the Victoria Jackson Cosmetics line.

Free radical. An atom or molecule with an unpaired electron that is highly unstable and damaging to other molecules. In skin tissue, free radicals contribute to aging. Free radicals are neutralized by antioxidants. Smoking creates free radicals, reduces the delivery of oxygen to the skin, and causes rapid aging of the skin.

Fun basket. A place to keep makeup for special occasions: it should contain all glittery and shiny makeup items, all dramatic and wild tones suitable for fun events only.

Glycerin. An odorless, colorless, syrupy liquid called a *humectant*. A humectant attracts water and hydrates chapped skin. Glycerin is used in skin moisturizers.

Hyperpigmentation. A skin condition characterized by brownish, dark-toned blotches. It can be caused by pregnancy, sun exposure, scarring, or cosmetic surgery procedures such as laser resurfacing and dermabrasion.

Lip balm. A stick, gel, or cream used to condition and heal chapped or dry lips. Lip balm commonly contains emollients, or softening agents. Cocoa butter, coconut oil, lanolin, petrolatum, and mineral oil are commonly used emollients. Lip balm also can contain aloe vera, vitamin E, antibacterial products such as tea tree oil, and sunblocks. Nonwaxy lip balms can be applied over lip color.

Lip cream. Colored pigment mixed with oils, polymers, wax, and vitamins. Lip creams, versus lipstick, offer the widest color selection and smoothest application to produce a classic, rich, moist opaque mouth.

Lip gloss and semi-gloss. Sheer or translucent colors in an oil or gel base. Semi-gloss products usually come in sticks. Lip gloss is commonly available in pots or wands.

Lip lacquer. Mouth color in a gel-based formula, available in pots. Lacquer delivers sheer color and a modest shine.

Lip liner. Pigments in pencil form used to outline the perimeter of the lips. However, creating a clearly defined line or lining the lips in a dark or contrasting color is no longer fashionable. In the new millennium, lip liner is used to contour, shape, and balance lips, then blended into the lip color. Liner also helps keep lip color from bleeding into fine mouth lines.

Lip satin. Colors made from oils and polymers that lubricate the lips, leaving a finish somewhere between a matte and a gloss.

Lip stain. Dyes that stain the lips, giving a dry finish that actually changes natural lip color for a period of time.

Lipstick. Colors for the mouth made of waxes, oils, dyes, and various added ingredients including polymers, silicones, vitamins, and sun screens. Red pigment can actually stain the natural lips if used on a constant basis.

Mascara. Brown or black pigments (other colors occasionally used) in a base of water, alcohol, waxes, glycerin, and other ingredients. Mascara is applied with a wand or brush to darken, lengthen, thicken, and condition eyelashes. It is packaged in a cake, water soluble, waterproof, or clear form.

Matte. A skin surface or makeup product without shine. Matte lipsticks are made from volatile silicones that instantly evaporate, leaving pigments and waxes in a no-shine, long-lasting coverage.

Melasma or mask of pregnancy. Hyperpigmentation of skin caused by hormonal changes during pregnancy resulting in brown or dark blotches on the face. Women with dark hair and eyes are more prone to this condition. *See* **Hyperpigmentation**.

Moisturizer. An emollient that provides a barrier between the skin and air to keep moisture from absorbing. Moisturizers contain various oils, vitamins, humectants, and water, commonly combined with a fragrance and coloring in a lotion, gel, or cream form. The newest moisturizers add alpha-hydroxy or glycolic acids which not only exfoliate the skin, but help deliver antioxidants, such as vitamin C, or skin rejuvenating substances, such as collagen and elastin, to deeper layers of the dermis.

Oil absorbers. Kaolin and/or talc added to makeup to absorb excess facial oil and give the skin a matte appearance.

Oil-control blotting paper. Small swatches of paper containing powder. Economical and easy-to-carry in a purse, they help reduce shine on the face throughout the day or evening.

Overcorrected lips. Drawing lip liner beyond the outside edge of the lips. Instead of making the lips look fuller, this practice simply draws attention to the problem being corrected.

Pay-off. A term referring to the incorrect application of powder, when too much pigment is deposited unequally. The cause is a poor puff which does not absorb the powder and leaves clumps on the face.

Powder. Talc or other oil-absorbing material placed on the skin or over foundation to absorb shine and any excess oils, not to apply color. A neutral-toned translucent powder applied with a compact-style puff is preferred.

Prom purse. Teenager's makeup bag containing a lipstick, lip gloss, blush, foundation, eye pencil, and waterproof mascara.

Retin-A (Tretinoin). A vitamin-derived solution available by prescription only. It diminishes fine lines and may retard the aging progress. It also is effective against acne.

Reverse raccoon eyes. A white mask around the eyes created by using a too light foundation to hide dark circles. This accentuates and draws attention to the problem.

Shimmer. Shine or glitter effect in eye shadow, blush, or body shimmer usually created by mica.

SPF. Skin Protection Factor. This rating is applied to sunscreens and sunblocks to indicate the amount of protection from sunlight offered by the product. Ratings between the ranges of SPF 15 and SPF 30 are optimal. The FDA suggests that over SPF 30, the extra protection is negligible. Premium lipsticks often contain SPF 25.

Stipling. A technique for applying foundation to the face utilizing dabs of color rather than a stroking application. Small dots or dabs of color will provide extra coverage without caking or a pancake look.

Tattooing. Permanent application of pigment into the skin. Tattooing is used primarily on the face to replace lost eyebrow hair. Another cosmetic use is the creation of permanent eyeliner, which is helpful to women who find the application of eyeliner difficult. Tattooing may be occasionally used to widen the appearance of the lips.

Transfer-resistant lipstick. Mouth color made from volatile silicones that vaporize and set the color. This color does not smear and lasts six to eight hours.

T-zone. The facial area encompassing the forehead, nose, and chin. Often oily skin is confined to this area, while other parts of the face are normal or dry.

Under-eye circles. Varying in color from brownish to blue, they are caused by veins visible through the skin or by darker skin pigmentation, a trait that is usually hereditary. Victoria Jackson recommends using eye cream to smooth out the skin texture, and then adding concealer. Too light a concealer can cause "reverse raccoon eyes."

Wide-set eyes. A term used to describe a larger than usual space between the inside corners and the bridge of the nose.

INDEX

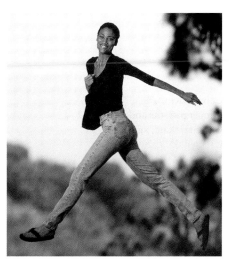

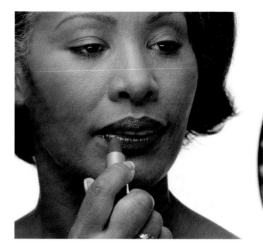

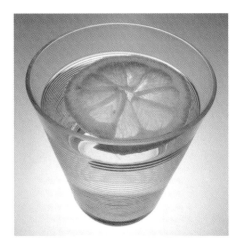